WEIGHT WATCHERS *FREESTYLE* COOKBOOK

The Complete Freestyle Smart Points Guide and 7 days meal plan for 2018

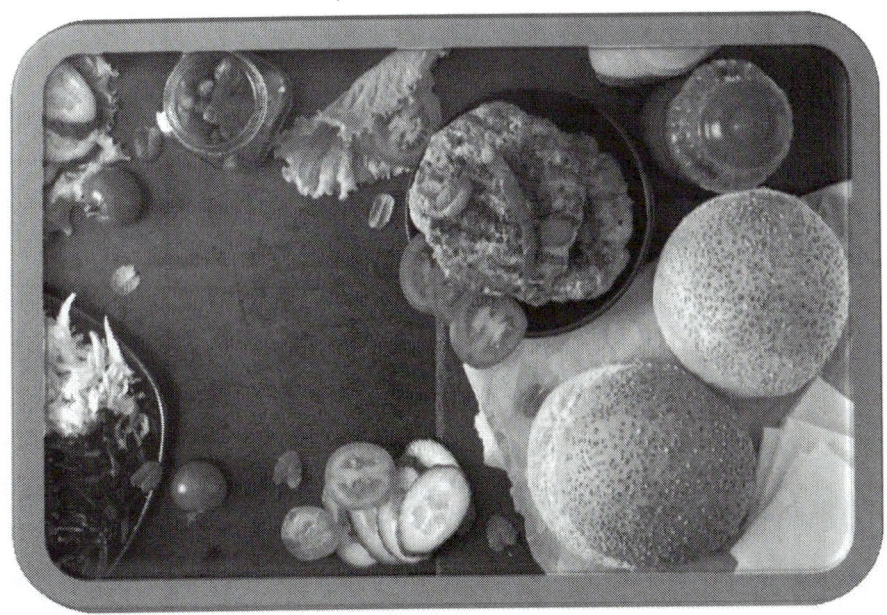

By Jamie Hayes

© Copyright 2018 by Jamie Hayes All rights reserved.

The following eBook is reproduced below with the goal of providing information that is as accurate and as reliable as possible. Regardless, purchasing this eBook can be seen as consent to the fact that both the publisher and the author of this book are in no way experts on the topics discussed within, and that any recommendations or suggestions made herein are for entertainment purposes only. Professionals should be consulted as needed before undertaking any of the action endorsed herein.

This declaration is deemed fair and valid by both the American Bar Association and the Committee of Publishers Association and is legally binding throughout the United States.

Furthermore, the transmission, duplication or reproduction of any of the following work, including precise information, will be considered an illegal act, irrespective whether it is done electronically or in print. The legality extends to creating a secondary or tertiary copy of the work or a recorded copy and is only allowed with express written consent of the Publisher. All additional rights are reserved.

The information in the following pages is broadly considered a truthful and accurate account of facts, and as such, any inattention, use or misuse of the information in question by the reader will render any resulting actions solely under their purview. There are no scenarios in which the publisher or the original author of this work can be in any fashion deemed liable for any hardship or damages that may befall them after undertaking information described herein.

Additionally, the information found on the following pages is intended for informational purposes only and should thus be considered, universal. As befitting its nature, the information presented is without assurance regarding its continued validity or interim quality. Trademarks that mentioned are done without written consent and can in no way be considered an endorsement from the trademark holder.

Table of Contents

Introduction 7
Weight Watchers 10
   The Program 10
   FreeStyle 2018 12
Freestyle Breakfast Recipes 13
   Freestyle Pimento Chile Chicken 14
   Zero Points Breakfast Pancakes 15
   Another Egg Muffin with 0 POINTS 15
   Salsa Roasted Salmon 16
   Scrambled Eggs with Spinach 17
   Healthy Oats and Peanut Butter 18
   Delicious Breakfast Casserole 18
   Ham and Egg Sandwich 19
   Egg and Ham Muffins 20
   Bacon and Zucchini Egg-Muffin 21
   Creamy-Tomato-Basil-Soup 22
   Chicken Taco Soup Recipe 23
   Tasty Slow Cooker Chili 24
   Vanilla Cinnamon Rolls 25
   Garlic Rice & Mushroom Risotto 26
   Roasted Sweet Potato Side Dish 27
   Apple Cheddar Turkey Wraps 28
   Cheesy, Twisty Ham Bread 30
   Tomato and Fresh Herb Frittata 31
   Chicken Stuffed Peppers 31
   Gravy and Biscuit Bake 32
   Egg Salad Sandwich 33
   Egg Muffin with Broccoli-Cheddar 34
   Freestyle One Pot Garlicky Cuban Pork 35
   Zero Points Bean Soup: 36

Tomato Spinach Soup 37
Mouth Watering Healthy Morning Cookies................................... 38
Delicious Instant Steamed Rice 39
Tasty Freestyle Butter Chicken Pot Pasta 40
Cinnamon-Apple French Toast 42
Zucchini and Corn Frittata.. 43
Baked Veggie-Egg Italian Style 44
Ham & Apricot Dijon Glaze... 45
Yummy Cheeseburger Soup 46
Heavenly Pancakes 47

Freestyle Lunch Recipes 48

Grilled Turkey Kebabs 49
Hawaiian Chicken Kebab... 49
Cilantro Lime Chicken Kabobs... 50
Potato-Crusted Butter and Herb Tilapia 51
Lemon Garlic Chicken and Asparagus 52
Delicious Pressure Cooker Texas Red Chili................................... 53
Tasty Turkey Meatball & Veggie 54
GreekStyle Chickpea Salad.. 56
Tasty Freestyle Buffalo Wing Hummus 57
Yummy Mediterranean Bean Salad... 57
Heavenly Apple Muffin 58
Sweet and Sour Meatballs 59
One Pan Shrimp Fajitas 60
Spaghetti Squash with Shrimps 61
Savory Chicken Dump Soup.. 62
Chicken Marsala MeatBall 63
Bruschetta Topped Balsamic Chicken.. 64
Scrumptious Pork chops and cabbage.. 66
Irresistible Freestyle White Chicken Chili 67
Watermelon, Jicama, & Cucumber Salad................................... 68
Delicious Mushroom and Spinach Quiche 69
Salmon with Garlic Zucchini Noodles 69
Easy Turkey Chili... 70
Tasty Whole Chicken in an Instant Pot 71

Freestyle Dinner Recipes 72

Delicious Pressure Cooker Red Beans and Rice 73
Chicken Marsala Meatballs... 75
Simple Vegan Potato Soup.. 76
African Sweet Potato Stew... 77
Slow Cooker Chicken and Tomato Orzo 78

Tasty Turkey Meatball & Veggie Soup 79
Sticky Buffalo Chicken Tenders 80
Slow Cook Chicken Cacciatore 81
Garlic Roasted Garbanzo Beans.. 83
Sea Scallops, Arugula, & Beet Salad.. 84
Scrumptious Cheese and Ham Omelet... 85
Heavenly Beans & Vegan Nachos In the Pot 85
Freestyle Corn & Zucchini Summer Frittata.. 86
Spiralized Apple & Cabbage Slaw... 87
Lentil and Vegetable Stew.. 88
Beef Italian Soup 89
Greek Lemon Chicken Soup 90
Turkey Vegetable Soup 91
Sweet & Sour Turkey Meatballs 92
Tasty BBQ Apricot Chicken.. 93
Pizza Lasagna Roll-Ups... 93
Delicious Crispy Apple Surprise.. 95
Tasty Pressure cooked beef ribs... 96
Freestyle Ham and Cheese Egg Cups... 97
Heavenly Low Yolk Egg Salad 98
Sticky Buffalo Chicken Tenders 98
Chicken Fried Rice 99
Irresistible Potato and Cheese Casserole... 100

Freestyle Soup Recipes 101

Chicken & Veggie Soup 101
Cod & Quinoa Soup 102
Chicken & Lime Soup.. 103
Meatballs & Kale Soup.. 104
Beef & Veggies Soup... 105
Ground Beef Soup 106
Meatballs & Zucchini Soup 107
Chicken & Zucchini Soup.. 108
Pork & Veggie Soup 109
Salmon Soup... 110
Veggies Soup 111
Barley & Chickpeas Soup 112
Chicken & Greens Soup.. 113
Rice Noodles & Veggie Soup 114

Snack & Appetizer Recipes... 115

Roasted Almonds applesauce... 115
Tasty Roasted Chickpeas 116

Hot & Spicy Popcorn	116
Salt And Pepper Spinach Chips	117
Bake Kale Chips	117
Hot Pepper Apple Chips	118
Ginger Parsnip Fries	119
Roasted Pumpkin Seeds	119
Roasted Cashews	120
Russet Potato Fries	120
Cauliflower Poppers	121
Quinoa Croquettes	121
Coconut Chicken Popcorn	122
Butter Currant Biscuits	123
Green Deviled Eggs	124
Tomato Bruschetta	124
Vanilla Almond Scones	125
Blueberry Balls Cookie	126
Bonus The Best Smart Points Main course Recipes	**127**
Honey Sesame Chicken	128
Chicken Fried Rice	129
Tasty Orange Chicken	130
Cajun Chicken and Sweet Potato Hash	131
Spiced Pork with Apples	132
Pork Chops with Salsa	133
Italian Steak Rolls	134
Beef Soba Bowls	135
Baked Artichoke Chicken	136
Slow Cooker Spiced Pulled Pork	137
Curried Pork Chops	138
Spicy Pineapple Pork	139
Breaded Veal Cutlets	140
Cheesy Fajita Casserole	141
Creamy Dijon Chicken	142
Grilled Chicken Salad	143
Delicious Chicken Salad	144
Raspberry Balsamic Chicken	145

Introduction

The reasons why people lose weight vary from person to person. Over the past two decades, obesity has greatly increased in the USA with statistics showing that more than a third of adults in the USA are overweight. When one is overweight, he or she has a lot of physiological as well as emotional issues, hence people having varied reasons for wanting to lose weight:

- **Being Healthy**

During a research carried out in 2007, half of the target population said their major reason for losing weight was to improve their health. When obese, one is at a risk of developing heart disease, stroke as well as cancer.

- **Mood**

Why is this so? When one is overweight, he or she has insecurities that lead to depression as well as low self-esteem. Moreover, there is also some evidence that disorders related to one's mood and obesity is connected. Also, depression and bipolar disorder may be a precursor to obesity. Past studies have also proved that losing weight leads to improved mood.

- **Fitness**

This is true especially for men who are regarded as being overweight.

- **Wanting to have children**

This is because being overweight can lead to infertility and other complications during pregnancy. As we delve further into weight loss, the amount of weight you need to shed isn't really an important thing as such. You really need to know your real reasons for wanting to lose weight. We may have several reasons for wanting to shed weight, but we may not really realize what they are. When people are asked why they need to lose weight, most of them say: they want to be fit and healthy, they want to be confident, respected, love and so forth.

Consequently, you may start feeling trapped by your weight. You will start being obsessed about what you eat and the amount of exercise you do. There may be people who are leaner than you, but they are less confident, feel less loved and respected. Please be careful to lose weight for the correct reasons. If you have some solid reason for losing weight, you will definitely stick to your diet plan. There are good reasons as well as bad reasons for losing weight. The bad reasons may make you lose weight, but they will not be good enough for a long-term change in one's habits and lifestyle.

Good reasons for losing weight revolve around you while the negative ones revolve around pleasing other people such as:

- Shedding weight so as to attract someone

This may be a great trigger for weight loss; looking nice for someone you would want to be with. However, ask yourself what happens if this person does not exist in your life anymore? You will definitely lose your motivation for losing weight.

- Weight loss to boost health

This will be about you and it does not depend on what someone else thinks, says or does.

- Being referred to as overweight

Insults could motivate you to change your appearance. However, you don't need to change so as to impress someone.

In short, losing weight needs to be about you and nobody else. This is the only way to maintain your motivation and be focused on your goals.

Many people, including you, who is reading this, don't understand the main reasons why they want to lose weight. Your reasons for weight loss should be deeper and meaningful; they need to originate from your inner self. As soon as you have your valid reasons for losing weight, jot them down on an index card. Place them by your bedside and read them when you wake up and before retiring to bed.

Furthermore, you can also keep a copy at work and another in your wallet as a constant reminder of your goals. You should also know that weight-loss goals, determine the difference between success and failure. Goals that are well-planned will keep you focused and motivated. Goals that are not realistic and overly ambitious will definitely undermine your efforts. Below are tips on losing weight:

- Concentrate on process goals

An outcome goal could be what you hope to achieve in the end. Even though this goal may give you a target, it does not guide you on how to achieve it. A process goal is a vital step in achieving whatever you desire. For instance, a process goal could be eating five portions of fruits or veggies on a daily basis, walking for half an hour daily or maybe drinking water after every meal. Process goals are particularly helpful when losing weight because you will focus on changing behaviors and habits that are important in weight loss.

- Set smart goals
1. They need to be specific- a good goal needs to have specific details.

2. They need to be measurable- if you can measure a goal, then you can objectively determine how successful you are at achieving the goal.
3. They need to be achievable- For instance, if your schedule doesn't allow you to spend an hour at the gym, then this is an unattainable goal.
4. They need to be realistic
- Your goals also need to be track-able
- Have long-term and short-term goals
- Don't try to be perfect

Setbacks are a natural part of behavior change. No one who is successful has never experienced setbacks. Identify potential barriers.

- Reassess and adjust goals as required

Weight Watchers
The Program

People used to strive for ways to find food. As the world advanced, we have so much of food that we don't know how to stop consuming it. That's where diet programs come in. The market is now congested with different dietary programs, all making claims of being the best. But few have achieved the heights that Weight Watchers has. And to know the secret behind Weight Watchers success we take an in-depth look into what makes it stand out.

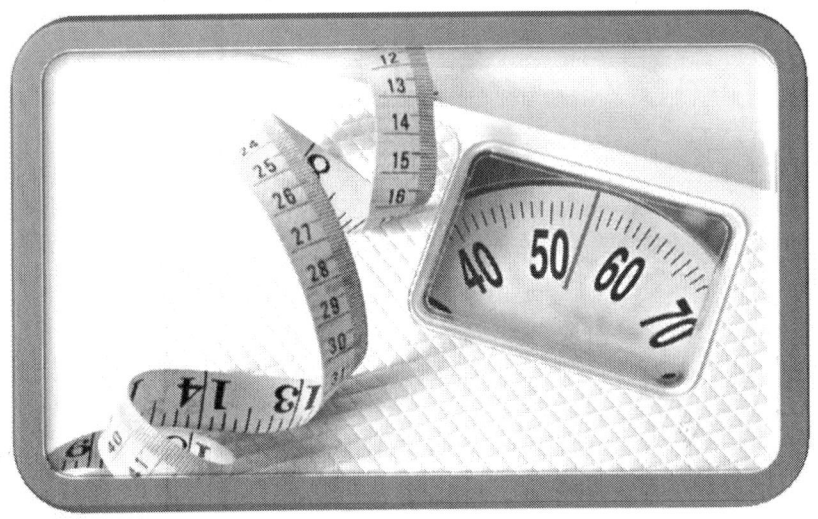

Evolution is what has kept us human beings the dominating creature. And this precise idea is what Weight Watchers have used to keep them on top. Weight Watchers introduces new and different ways to deal with so many of our daily problems. People who cannot attend meetings for any certain reasons can make use of the online forums, message boards and support groups. The newly introduced point system is also an example of how easy they make dieting for people who do not have time to calculate every single calorie they are consuming. The website itself is a dieter's heaven having everything an honest dieter would need to keep him in check and informed.

Weight Watchers is a great dieting program that is going to help you to lose weight in a safe and effective way. While other diet programs focus on really limiting your calories and telling you what you are allowed to eat and what you should stay away from. While this may work for some people, it can be a big challenge to always be kept away from some of their favourite foods. Plus making food purchases can be difficult on some of the diet plans.

Weight Watchers is going to work a bit differently. It realizes that you have a lot going on in life and you won't be able to sit around and purchase expensive products or go after hard to find ingredients in order to stay healthy. This one is based on the Smart Points that will allow you to eat the foods that work the best for you, but it does reward the healthy foods and discourages the unhealthy foods.

This plan is all about being conscious about your personal eating choices. You will be given a certain amount of points that you are able to use each day, and you get to choose how you use them up. Each of the foods that you choose will have a different point value assigned to it, and you can even make your own recipes and figure out the point values.

This program does allow you to have a bit of cheating throughout the week if you are really craving it or you are not able to resist for a big party. You will find that you can place these into your points values for the day and still eat them. As long as you are smart about some of the choices that you are making for the rest of the day, these little cheats are not going to ruin the hard work that you put in.

In addition to worrying about the healthy foods that you should consume during the week, there are other parts that come with Weight Watchers. These include going to the meetings and getting more activity into your daily life.

FreeStyle 2018

Based on the successful SmartPoints® system, WW Freestyle offers more than 200 zero Points® foods—including eggs, skinless chicken breast, fish and seafood, corn, beans, peas, and so much more—to multiply your meal and menu possibilities. And it makes life simpler, too: You can forget about weighing, measuring, or tracking those zero Points foods.

Freestyle Breakfast Recipes

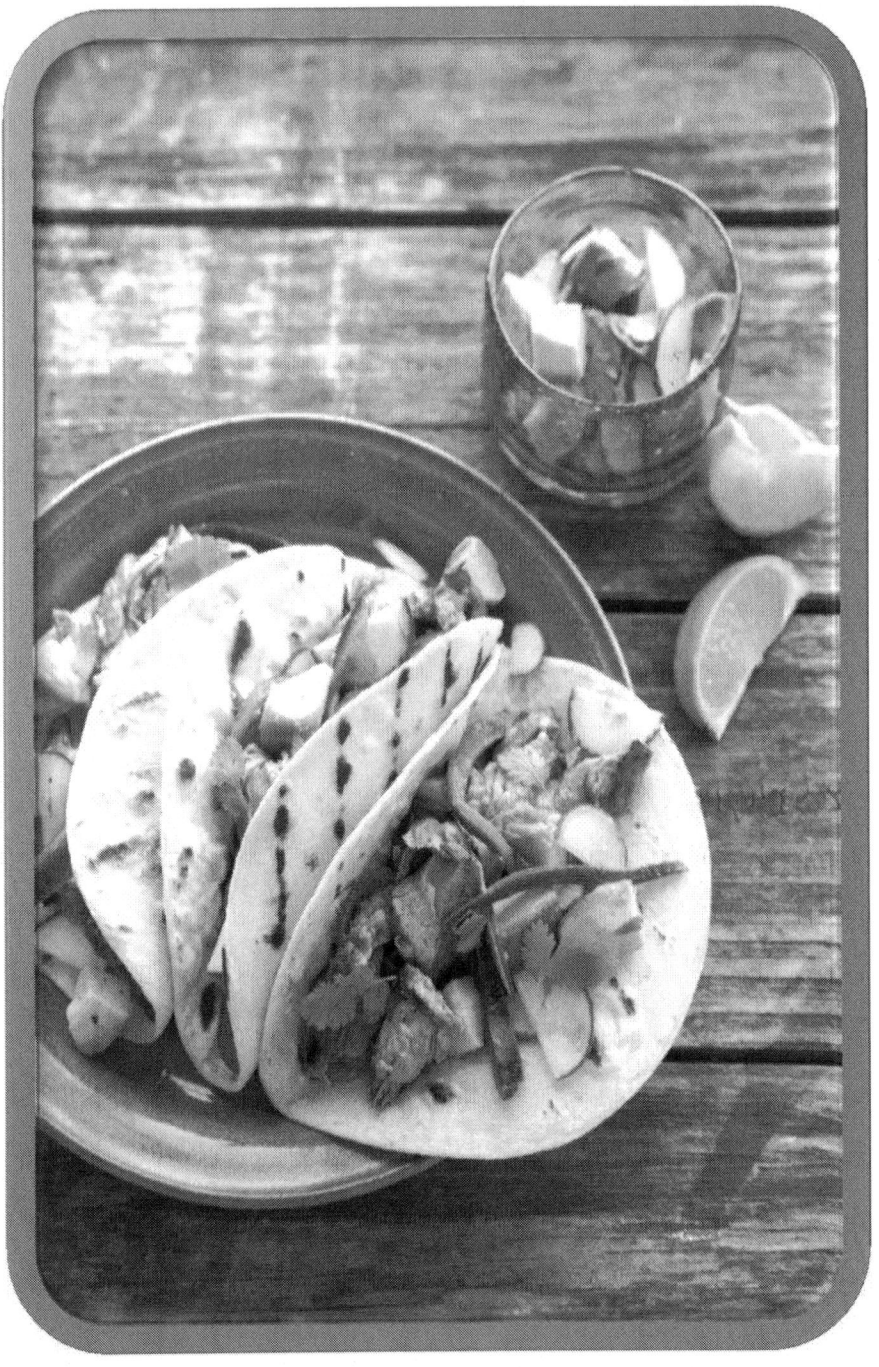

Freestyle Pimento Chile Chicken

Ingredients:
- 2 ½ c. cooked, chopped chicken breast (chopped into about 1/2" cubes
- ½ c. fat free chicken broth
- 1 ½ c. 98% fat free cream of mushroom soup (I use Campbell's)
- 1 ½ c. Healthy Request Condensed cream of chicken soup
- 1 4-oz. jar pimentos, drained (1/2 c.)
- 2 4-oz. cans Hatch green chiles, chopped and drained (You can add a 3rd can if you're just crazy about chiles like I am.)
- 10 oz. 50% reduced fat sharp cheddar cheese
- 6 oz. of Doritos (by weight) toasted corn tortilla chips, slightly crushed
- Pickled jalapeños, green onions, and/or cherry tomatoes for serving (optional)

Instructions:
1. Mix all ingredients except Doritos and cheese. In a large casserole dish (I use 9" x 13"), layer ½ of chicken mixture, then ½ of cheese, then ½ of the Doritos.
2. Repeat the same layers once more, ending with Doritos on top. Bake at 350° for about 40-45 minutes.
3. Cover top with foil if Doritos begin to brown too much. Serve with pickled jalapeños and/or your favorite salsa.

Makes 3 servings
3 SmartPoints per serving on FreeStyle Plan, and Flex Plan

Zero Points Breakfast Pancakes

Servings Per Recipe: 4, FREESTYLE POINTS: 0
Cooking Time: 5 minutes

Ingredients:
- ¼ tsp cinnamon
- 1 tsp vanilla
- 1 tsp baking powder
- 1 banana, mashed well
- 2 egg whites

Directions:
1. Place a griddle on medium fire and heat for at least 3 minutes.
2. In a medium bowl, whisk well egg whites.
3. Stir in cinnamon, vanilla, and baking powder.
4. Add mashed banana and mix thoroughly.
5. Evenly divide batter into 4 and cook for 2 minutes, flip and cook for half a minute. Repeat process for remaining batter.
6. Serve and enjoy with fresh berries.

Another Egg Muffin with 0 POINTS

Servings Per Recipe: 12, Freestyle Points: 0
Cooking Time: 40 minutes

Ingredients:
- ¼ tsp marjoram
- ¼ tsp red pepper flakes
- ½ tsp black pepper
- ½ tsp salt
- ½ tsp sage
- ½-lb 99% fat-free ground turkey breast

- 1 green bell pepper, diced
- 1 tsp Montreal Steak seasoning blend
- 12 eggs

Directions:
1. Place a nonstick skillet on medium-high fire and lightly grease with cooking spray.
2. Preheat oven to 350°F and lightly grease muffin tins with cooking spray.
3. Add ground turkey on skillet and sauté. Season with marjoram, red pepper flakes, black pepper, salt, and sage. Mix well and cook for 8 minutes or until no longer pink.
4. Meanwhile, in a bowl, whisk well the eggs and season with steak seasoning blend and stir in diced bell pepper. Combine thoroughly.
5. Once ground turkey is done cooking, evenly divide into the 12 muffin tins.
6. Pour egg mixture on top of ground turkey.
7. Pop in the oven and for 30 minutes bake.
8. Serve and enjoy.

Salsa Roasted Salmon

Servings Per Recipe: 2, POINTS: 0
Cooking Time: 15 minutes

Ingredients:
- 1 plum tomato, chopped
- ½ small onion, chopped
- 1 clove of garlic, minced
- Small jalapeno pepper, chopped
- 1 tsp apple cider vinegar
- ½ tsp chili powder
- ¼ tsp ground cumin

- ¼ tsp salt
- 3 dashes of Tabasco hot sauce
- 2 4-ounce salmon fillets

Directions:
1. Preheat the oven to 400°F.
2. In a food processor, mix the all the Ingredients: except for the salmon fillets. Blend until well combined.
3. Place the salmon in a roasting pan and pour the salsa on top.
4. Place inside the oven and roast for 15 minutes or until the salmon gets flaky.

Scrambled Eggs with Spinach

Servings Per Recipe: 6, POINTS: 1
Cooking Time: 10 minutes

Ingredients:
- 1 ½ tbsp. extra virgin olive oil
- ½ cup 2% sharp cheddar cheese
- 1 tsp salt
- 1 tsp pepper
- 1 clove garlic, crushed and minced
- ½ red onion, diced
- 3 cups organic baby spinach
- 1 organic tomato, diced
- 6 large eggs

Directions:
1. Whisk well salt, pepper, and eggs in a large bowl.
2. Place a large nonstick skillet on medium high fire and add oil. Heat for a minute.

3. Sauté garlic and onions for 5 minutes. Stir in tomatoes and sauté for 3 minutes.
4. Stir in spinach and cook for 2 minutes or until starting to wilt.
5. Pour in eggs and cook for 5 minutes, occasionally stirring.
6. Serve and enjoy.

Healthy Oats and Peanut Butter

Servings Per Recipe:1 , POINTS: 7
Prep Time: 5 minutes

Ingredients:
- 1 tbsp. sugar free jam
- 1 tbsp. peanut butter
- ¾ cup almond milk
- ½ cup old-fashioned oats

Directions:
1. In a bowl with lid, mix all Ingredients: except for the jam.
2. Cover and set in the fridge overnight.
3. Enjoy with a tablespoon of jam.

Delicious Breakfast Casserole

Servings Per Recipe: 6, POINTS: 5
Cooking Time: 50 minutes

Ingredients:
- 1 cup light grated cheese, divided
- ¾ cup diced onion
- 1 cup diced peppers
- 8-oz diced cooked ham
- 1 cup skim milk
- 3 egg whites
- 5 eggs

- 1 7.5-oz package Pillsbury biscuits

Directions:
1. Preheat oven to 350ºF and grease a 9x13-inch casserole dish.
2. Spread Pillsbury biscuits evenly on bottom of dish.
3. In a large bowl, whisk well eggs and egg whites.
4. Pour in milk and mix well.
5. Add onion, peppers, ham, and 2/3 cup of cheese. Whisk to combine and pour on top of biscuits.
6. Cover dish with foil and bake for 30 minutes.
7. Uncover and spread cheese on top and bake uncovered for another 15-20 minutes or until top is set and cheese is starting to brown.
8. Serve and enjoy while hot.

Ham and Egg Sandwich

Servings Per Recipe: 2, POINTS: 5
Cooking Time: 10 minutes

Ingredients:
- 4 tbsp. shredded asiago cheese, divided
- 4-oz deli ham
- 1 tbsp. ranch dressing
- A dash of paprika
- Pepper and salt to taste
- 1 tbsp. milk
- 1 egg white
- 1 egg
- 2 everything flat-out fold it bread

Directions:

1. Pick a bowl that can fit your bread in and whisk well paprika, pepper, salt, milk, egg white, and eggs.
2. Place a medium nonstick frypan on medium fire and let it heat.
3. Meanwhile, spread dressing over each fold and add 2 tbsp. of cheese and 2-oz of ham on each bread.
4. Dip bread in bowl of egg, thoroughly and place in pan.
5. Cook for 5 minutes and turnover and cook for another 5 minutes.
6. Serve and enjoy.

Egg and Ham Muffins

Servings Per Recipe: 12, POINTS: 3
Cooking Time: 20 minutes

Ingredients:
- Paprika, pepper, and salt to taste
- 12 eggs
- 12 slices of ham, no preservatives

Directions:
1. Preheat oven to 375°F.
2. With ham, line muffin tin with 1 ham each.
3. Break the eggs one at a time with one egg introduced inside the cupped ham.
4. Season each muffin with pepper, salt, and paprika to taste.
5. Pop in the oven and bake for 20 minutes.
6. Once done, serve and enjoy.

Bacon and Zucchini Egg-Muffin

Servings Per Recipe: 3
POINTS: 4
Cooking Time: 20 minutes

Ingredients:
- ½ cup shredded part skim mozzarella
- Pepper and salt to taste
- ¼ cup skim milk
- 6 egg whites
- 6 eggs
- 1 zucchini, diced
- 6 pieces turkey bacon, chopped

Directions:
1. With cooking spray, lightly grease muffin tin and preheat oven to 375°F.
2. Place a nonstick cooking pan on medium fire and lightly grease with cooking spray.
3. Add bacon to pan and sauté until crisped, around 6 minutes. Transfer bacon to a plate and discard bacon fat.
4. Add zucchini to pan and sauté until tender, around 5 minutes. Transfer to plate of bacon.
5. In a large bowl, whisk egg whites and eggs. Season with pepper and salt.
6. Stir in milk, cheese, cooked zucchini, and browned bacon.
7. Evenly divide into 6 muffin tins.
8. Pop in the oven and bake for 20 minutes.
9. Serve and enjoy.

Creamy-Tomato-Basil-Soup

Serves: 4

Ingredients

- 1 cup low sodium chicken broth (or vegetable broth if you prefer)
- 1 14 oz. can tomato puree
- 1 cup skim milk
- 4-5 leaves fresh basil
- 3 tsp. olive oil
- 1 stalk celery
- ½ cup onions
- 1 Tbsp. cornstarch
- 1-2 cloves garlic, crushed.
- pepper to taste

Instructions

1. Rough chop onions and celery, transfer them to a food processor or chopper and puree until fine.
2. Heat olive oil in a large pan over medium heat.
3. Add onion and celery mix to pan and sauté until they begin to become translucent.
4. Reduce heat to low and stir in garlic, pepper, chicken stock, and tomato puree, and cornstarch-simmer on low for 5 minutes.
5. Whisk in tomato puree and milk, top with basil leaves, simmer for an additional 10 minutes.
6. Serve topped with a dollop of Greek yogurt or a fresh chopped basil.
7. This makes approximately 4 -1/2 cup servings

Makes 2 large servings
5 SmartPoints per serving on FreeStyle Plan, and Flex Plan

Chicken Taco Soup Recipe

Prep time:5 m, Cook time:30 m, Total time:35 m
Serves: 8

Ingredients
- 2 Cups Shredded or Cubed Chicken
- 1 onion, diced
- 1 bell pepper, diced
- 1 poblano pepper, diced
- 2 tomatoes, chopped
- 1 tablespoon garlic, minced
- 6 cups fat free chicken broth
- 1 cup tomato sauce
- 1½ cups kidney beans or pinto beans
- 2 tablespoons taco/fajita seasoning
- 1 tablespoon olive oil

Instructions
1. In a large stockpot, sauté the onion, bell pepper, poblano pepper, and tomato for 5 minutes stirring regularly. You want the vegetables to be tender.
2. Mix in chicken, broth, tomato sauce, garlic, pinto beans, and seasonings.
3. Simmer on medium heat for 30 minutes, stirring occasionally.
4. Serve with preferred garnishes like cheese, sour cream, or tortilla chips.

WW Information:
Makes 8 Servings (approximately 2 cups each)
3 SmartPoints per serving on
1 Smart Point per serving on FreeStyle Plan or FlexPlan

Tasty Slow Cooker Chili

COOKING TIME: 4-5 hours
SERVES: 6
POINTS: 4
INGREDIENTS:
½ pound extra lean ground beef or turkey,
1 medium green bell pepper (deseeded, diced),
1 medium red bell pepper (deseeded, diced),
1 teaspoon garlic (minced),
14 ounces canned crushed tomatoes,
2 tablespoons canned diced green chilies or 1 small jalapeño pepper (sliced),
7.5 ounces canned kidney beans (drained, rinsed),
1 teaspoon ground cumin,
1 tablespoon chili powder,
1 small onion (chopped),
Salt to taste,
Pepper to taste
And 1 tablespoon tomato paste
INSTRUCTIONS:
1) Place a skillet over medium heat. Add beef and garlic and sauté until brown. Break it simultaneously as it cooks. Add bell peppers and sauté for a couple of minutes. Add cumin and chili powder and stir.
2) Transfer into the slow cooker. Add rest of the ingredients and stir well.
3) Cover and cook on 'High' for 4-5 hours. Ladle into bowls and serve.

Vanilla Cinnamon Rolls

Ingredients:
- ¼ c. cream cheese
- ¼ c. sugar
- ¼ tsp. vanilla
- 1 tsp. butter, melted
- 11 oz. breadstick dough, cold
- 2 Tbsp. brown sugar
- 1 tsp. cinnamon

Directions:
1. Turn on the oven and let it heat up to 375 degrees. While that is heating up, take out a baking pan and prepare it with some cooking spray.
2. Take out a small bowl and mix together the brown sugar, cinnamon, and the butter and place to the side.
3. Take the breadstick dough and make it into 12 strips. Sprinkle on some brown sugar to this dough and then roll them into a spiral. Press the dough down to seal up the ends.
4. Place these rolls into a baking pan, leaving them about an inch apart. Place into the oven and let them bake for 15 minutes. When they are done, take out of the oven and let them cool for 10 minutes.
5. While the rolls are baking, work on the frosting. Bring out a bowl and mix together the cream cheese, sugar, and vanilla. Add a bit of water to this until you get the consistency that you would like.
6. Drizzle this frosting onto the prepared rolls and let it set for a few minutes before serving.

Makes 2 large servings, 2 SmartPoints per serving on Beyond the Scale, FreeStyle Plan, and Flex Plan

Garlic Rice & Mushroom Risotto

Ready in 30 minutes,
5-6 servings
6 Points.

Ingredients
- 1/2 cup white onion, minced
- 4 cloves minced garlic
- 1 tablespoon olive oil
- 5 ounces' mushrooms, chopped into small pieces
- salt and thyme, 1 teaspoon each
- 3 cups vegetable broth
- 1 cup dry white wine
- 2 cups Arborio rice
- 1/2 cup lemon juice
- 3 cups fresh spinach
- 1 tablespoon vegan butter substitute
- 1 tablespoon nutritional yeast
- Black pepper

Instructions
1. Turn rice cooker and leave the lid open. Add the oil and let it heat.
2. Add the onions and garlic, stir gently to soften. Stir in the mushrooms, thyme and salt.
3. Add the wine and vegetable broth, stir continuously.
4. Add Arborio rice and stir well.
5. Cover the cooker tightly with lid and restart the cooking timer.
6. Allow rice cook as per the prescribed cycle, stir well when cooking is complete.

7. Transfer rice into a serving bowl. Stir in lemon juice, vegan butter substitute, spinach, nutritional yeast and black pepper until the butter substitute melts completely and all the rest of ingredients are well stirred together. Serve warm.

Nutrition information
Calories: 454.5
Carbohydrates: 36.4g
Fats: 15.2g
Proteins: 0g

Roasted Sweet Potato Side Dish

Prep time: 5 mins
Cook time: 25 mins
Total time: 30 mins

Ingredients
- 2 Medium Sweet Potatoes
- ½ teaspoon salt
- Non-Stick Cooking Spray

Instructions
1. Preheat oven to 400 degrees.
2. Line baking sheet with silicone baking mat or spray with non-stick spray.
3. Clean sweet potatoes, and peel if desired. We usually leave the skin intact. Remove any blemishes or eyes if needed.
4. Slice sweet potatoes into ¼" thick medallions
5. Place sweet potatoes in a single layer on prepared baking sheet.
6. Sprinkle the tops lightly with salt.

7. Bake at 400 degrees for 15 minutes. Turn sweet potato medallions over and bake additional 10 minutes.

This recipe makes 4 servings.
Each serving is approximately 1/2 sweet potato.
5 SmartPoints per serving on FreeStyle Plan or Flex Plan

Apple Cheddar Turkey Wraps

Yield: 1 WRAP

INGREDIENTS:
- 1 Flat-out Light Original Flatbread
- 1-2 leaves green leaf lettuce, torn
- 2 oz. thinly sliced deli turkey
- 1 oz. sliced 50% reduced fat sharp cheddar cheese
- 1 ½ teaspoons apple cider vinegar
- ½ teaspoon canola oil
- ½ teaspoon honey
- A pinch of salt and pepper
- ¼ cup matchstick-sliced apple pieces (slice apple into thin, short sticks)
- 1/3 cup coleslaw mix (just the shredded veggies, undressed)

DIRECTIONS:

1. Lay the Flat-out flatbread on a clean, dry surface and lay the torn lettuce down the center of the flatbread going the long way (starting at the rounded end and spreading down the length of the flatbread to the other rounded end). You can leave a bit of space at each end as you'll be folding them over, and you do not need to cover the whole flatbread, just an area down the middle. Top the lettuce with the sliced deli turkey and the cheddar cheese. *Make sure to leave an inch or so of room at each end.*
2. In a small mixing bowl, combine the vinegar, oil, honey, salt and pepper and stir until well combined. Add the apples and coleslaw and stir to coat. Lay the apple/coleslaw mixture on top of the other ingredients layered on the wrap.
3. Fold in the rounded ends of the flatbread over the filling. Then fold one of the long edges over the filling and continue to roll until the wrap is completely rolled up. Cut in half and serve.

WEIGHT WATCHERS FREESTYLE SMARTPOINTS:
7 per wrap
NUTRITION INFORMATION:
277 calories, 26 g carbs, 8 g sugars, 9 g fat, 3 g saturated fat, 28 g protein, 10 g fiber

Cheesy, Twisty Ham Bread

Servings Per Recipe: 12, POINTS: 3
Cooking Time: minutes

Ingredients:
- ¾ cup shredded 2% sharp cheddar cheese
- 4 tsps. mustard
- 6-oz deli ham
- 1 11-oz can of Pillsbury French Bread Crusty French Loaf dough

Directions:
1. Lightly grease a baking sheet with cooking spray and preheat oven to 350ºF.
2. Unroll dough to a flat rectangle. With a rolling pin, roll dough to an 11x15 rectangle. The cut the dough, in half lengthwise creating two pieces of 5.5x15-inch length dough.
3. On piece of dough, evenly spread the ham. Top with mustard and spread evenly. Then evenly spread cheese on top of mustard. Cover with the other dough and press edges with fingers to firmly seal sides.
4. With a pizza cutter, slice equally in 12 strips.
5. To twist the dough, hold one end of a strip and then twist the other side to desired number of twists. Place on prepared baking dish. Repeat process to remaining strips.
6. Pop in the oven and bake until dough is a golden brown, around 25 to 28 minutes.

Tomato and Fresh Herb Frittata

Servings Per Recipe: 4, POINTS: 7
Cooking Time: 20 minutes

Ingredients:
- 1/2cup crumpled goat cheese
- 1 cup cherry tomatoes, halved
- 1 tbsp. fresh parsley, chopped
- 2 tbsp. basil, chopped
- 2 tbsp. chives, chopped
- ¼ tsp freshly ground pepper
- ½ tsp salt
- ¼ cup 1% milk
- 8 large eggs

Directions:
1. Lightly grease a 9-inch round baking dish and preheat oven to 450of.
2. In a large bowl, whisk well pepper, salt, milk, and eggs.
3. In prepared dish, evenly spread herbs and tomatoes. Sprinkle cheese on top.
4. Pour egg mixture in baking dish.
5. Pop in the oven and bake for 20 minutes or until tops are set.
6. Evenly divide into 4, serve, and enjoy.

Chicken Stuffed Peppers

Servings Per Recipe: 4, POINTS: 3
Cooking Time: 35 minutes

Ingredients:
- 4 tbsp. shredded asiago cheese
- ¼ cup light ranch dressing
- 12-oz cooked, shredded chicken

- 1 tsp oil
- 1 red onion
- 4 large bell peppers of choice with tops cut and discarded, inside is hollowed out

Directions:
1. Preheat oven to 375oF.
2. On a baking dish, place peppers and bake for ten minutes to soften them.
3. Meanwhile, place a nonstick skillet on medium-high fire. Sauté onion for 8 minutes, until soft.
4. In a bowl, mix well ranch dressing, sautéed onions, and shredded chicken.
5. Once peppers are done baking, evenly stuff with the chicken mixture and return to oven.
6. Bake for 30 minutes.
7. When time is up, remove peppers, sprinkle cheese on top, and return to oven. Broil for 3 minutes.
8. Then serve and enjoy.

Gravy and Biscuit Bake

Servings Per Recipe: 6, POINTS: 7
Cooking Time: 30 minutes

Ingredients:
- 8-oz Jennie-O Lean Turkey Breakfast Sausage
- 1 pkg McCormick Country Gravy Mix, prepared with water
- 1 ½ cups egg beaters
- 1.75-oz can Pillsbury Buttermilk Biscuits
- 1 cup reduced fat mild cheddar

Directions:

1. Lightly grease a 9x13 baking dish with cooking spray and preheat oven to 350oF.
2. Place a nonstick skillet on medium-high fire and sauté turkey sausage until cooked, around 8 minutes. Discard fat and set aside.
3. Mix and cook the gravy mix according to package instructions.
4. Evenly spread the biscuits in bottom of baking dish.
5. Pour egg beaters on top and evenly spread sausage.
6. Pop in the oven and bake for 20 minutes.
7. Remove dish from oven and evenly sprinkle with cheese and return to oven.
8. Continue baking for another ten minutes.
9. Remove from oven, let it sit for 5 minutes before serving.

Egg Salad Sandwich

Servings Per Recipe: 5, POINTS: 3
Prep Time: 5 minutes

Ingredients:
- 10 slices light bread, toasted if desired
- 1 tsp sugar
- 1 tbsp. mustard
- 2 tbsp. tartar sauce
- 6 hard-boiled eggs

Directions:
1. In a medium bowl, mash hardboiled eggs with two forks.
2. Stir in sugar, mustard, and tartar sauce. Mix well.

3. On a piece of bread, spread ¼ cup of egg mixture, and then top with another slice of bread. Repeat process to remaining egg mixture and bread slices.
4. Serve and enjoy.

Egg Muffin with Broccoli-Cheddar

Servings Per Recipe: 6
POINTS: 4
Cooking Time: 15 minutes

Ingredients:
- 2 green onions, chopped
- ¾ cup reduced fat shredded cheddar cheese
- 2 cups broccoli, steamed and chopped
- Pepper and salt to taste
- ½ tbsp. Dijon mustard
- 4 egg whites
- 8 eggs

Directions:
1. Lightly grease muffin tins with cooking spray and preheat oven to 350°F.
2. In a bowl, whisk well pepper, salt, mustard, egg whites, and eggs.
3. Add cheddar cheese, green onions, and broccoli.
4. Evenly divide the mixture into 12 muffin tins.
5. Pop in the oven and bake for 13 minutes or until puffy and center is set.
6. Serve and enjoy.

Freestyle One Pot Garlicky Cuban Pork

5 Points

213 calories

TOTAL TIME: 80 minutes plus marinade time

INGREDIENTS:

- 3 lb. boneless pork shoulder blade roast, lean, all fat removed
- 6 cloves garlic
- juice of 1 grapefruit (about 2/3 cup)
- juice of 1 lime
- 1/2 tablespoon fresh oregano
- 1/2 tablespoon cumin
- 1 tablespoon kosher salt
- 1 bay leaf
- lime wedges, for serving
- chopped cilantro, for serving
- hot sauce, for serving
- tortillas, optional for serving
- salsa, optional for serving

DIRECTIONS:

1. Cut the pork in 4 pieces and place in a bowl.
2. In a small blender or mini food processor, combine garlic, grapefruit juice, lime juice, oregano, cumin and salt and blend until smooth.
3. Pour the marinade over the pork and let it sit room temperature 1 hour or refrigerated as long as overnight.
4. Transfer to the pressure cooker, add the bay leaf, cover and cook high pressure 80 minutes. Let the pressure release naturally.
5. Remove pork and shred using two forks.

6. Remove liquid from pressure cooker, reserving then place the pork back into pressure cooker. Add about 1 cup of the liquid (jus) back, adjust the salt as needed and keep warm until you're ready to eat.

NUTRITION INFORMATION
Yield: 10 servings,
Serving Size: a little over 3 oz.

Amount Per Serving:
- Smart Points: 5
- Calories: 213
- Total Fat: 9.5g
- Saturated Fat: 0g
- Cholesterol: 91mg
- Sodium: 440.5mg
- Carbohydrates: 2.5g
- Fiber: 0.5g
- Sugar: 1.5g
- Protein: 26.5g

Zero Points Bean Soup:

0 WW Freestyle Smart Points (12 approximately 1 cup servings)

Ingredients:
- 2 cans white beans (rinsed and drained)
- 2 cans Lima beans (rinsed and drained)
- 2 cans corn kernels drained
- 1 carton low sodium vegetable broth
- 12 slices Canadian Bacon chopped into small pieces
- Season to taste,

Directions:

1. Dump all ingredients into a large crockpot.
2. Stir gently to evenly mix ingredients.
3. Cook on low 6-8 hours. This is zero points...you have enough left for cornbread!

Tomato Spinach Soup

COOKING TIME: 4 hours, SERVES: 4, POINTS: 2
INGREDIENTS:
1 medium carrot (chopped),
5 ounces baby spinach,
1 medium stalk celery (chopped),
1 clove garlic (minced),
1 medium onion (chopped),
2 cups vegetable broth,
Salt to taste,
Pepper to taste,
½ teaspoon dried oregano
½ tablespoon dried basil,
¼ teaspoon crushed red pepper flakes,
14 ounces canned diced tomatoes
And 1 bay leaf
INSTRUCTIONS:
1) Add all the ingredients into the slow cooker. Clover and set on High for 5 hours.
2) Discard bay leaf and stir. Ladle into soup bowls and serve

Mouth Watering Healthy Morning Cookies

Ingredients:
2 egg whites
1/3 c. unsweetened cocoa
1/3 c. chocolate chips, mini
½ c. brown sugar, pressed down
½ c. sugar
1/8 tsp. salt
¼ c. butter, softened
1 c. flour
¼ tsp. baking soda

Directions:
1. Turn on the oven and let it heat up to 350 degrees. Take out a cookie sheet and spray it with some cooking spray.
2. Now take out a bowl and mix together the baking soda, flour, and salt. In a second bowl, combine the butter and the brown sugar and mix together until fluffy.
3. Add in the sugar to this second bowl and continue to beat to make it well incorporated. Put all of this into the flour mixture and keep on stirring to combine. Now add in the chocolate chips.
4. Place small amounts of this onto the cookie sheet and then put into the oven and let it bake for about 10 minutes.
5. Take out of the oven and allow the cookies to cool down for a few minutes before taking them off the pan and cooling down completely.

Delicious Instant Steamed Rice

Ready in 25 minutes,
4 servings.
5 Points.
Ingredients
- 1 cup Basmati or any long grain white rice
- 2 cups water
- 1 teaspoon olive oil

Instructions
1. Add the rice, water and oil to the pressure cooker. Cover cooker with lid.
2. Cook in high heat and high pressure. Lower the heat, maintain it and cook for up to 4 minutes.
3. Open the cooker with the natural release method. Transfer the cooker from the burner without removing the lid.
4. Instead, allow 10 minutes for the contents completely cook and steam. Fluff with a fork and serve.

Nutrition information
Calories: 199
Carbohydrates: 44.7g
Fats: 0.4g
Proteins: 4.2g

Tasty Freestyle Butter Chicken Pot Pasta

Yield: 8 (1 1/4 CUPS) SERVINGS
INGREDIENTS:
- 1 ½ lbs. uncooked boneless, skinless chicken breasts
- 4 tablespoons light butter
- ½ cup chopped onion
- ¼ cup flour
- ½ teaspoon salt
- ¼ teaspoon black pepper
- 1 ½ cups skim milk
- 2 ½ cups water*
- 1 tablespoon Better Than Bouillon Roasted Chicken Base
- ½ teaspoon poultry seasoning
- 8 oz. uncooked egg noodles
- 1 cup frozen corn kernels
- 2 cups frozen peas and carrots

DIRECTIONS:
1. Place the chicken breasts in a Dutch oven or other large pot and cover with water to about 2 inches over the chicken.
2. Bring the water to a boil over high heat and then reduce the heat to medium. Cook over medium heat for 15-20 minutes (depending on the thickness of your chicken breasts – mine are generally done at 15, so check one then) until chicken is cooked through.

3. Remove the chicken breasts to a cutting board. Discard the water from the pot and rinse and wipe out the pot to use again. Chop the chicken into small, bite-size pieces and set aside.
4. Melt the butter in the pot over medium heat. Add the chopped onion and cook for a few minutes until the onion is softened.
5. Whisk in the flour, salt and pepper until combined with the butter and onions and continue to whisk for another 1-2 minutes.
6. Slowly whisk in the milk until combined and smooth. Add the water and bouillon base (or broth) and poultry seasoning and whisk in to combine.
7. Increase the heat to med-high and stir occasionally until boiling. Reduce the heat to med-low and add the egg noodles. Cook for 8 minutes, stirring regularly to prevent sticking. If you need a little more liquid toward the end you can add a bit more water or broth.
8. Add the chopped chicken, corn, and peas and carrots and stir until thoroughly combined. Cook for another few minutes until all ingredients are heated through.

NUTRITION INFORMATION PER (1 ¼ CUP) SERVING: 314 calories, 35 g carbs, 3 g sugars, 7 g fat, 2 g saturated fat, 27 g protein, 3 g fiber

Cinnamon-Apple French Toast

Servings Per Recipe: 4
POINTS: 4
Cooking Time: 45 minutes

Ingredients:
- 1 cup 1% milk
- 1 1/3 cup liquid egg whites
- 4 eggs
- 2 tsps. cinnamon
- 2 apples, peeled and diced
- 8 slices low calorie bread

Directions:
1. Lightly grease a 9x13-inch casserole dish with cooking spray and preheat oven to 350°F.
2. In a microwave safe bowl, mix a tsp of cinnamon with diced apples and microwave for 3 minutes.
3. In prepared casserole dish, place bread slices and evenly top with cooked apples.
4. In a bowl, whisk well milk, egg whites, and eggs. Pour over bread in casserole dish.
5. Pop in the oven and cook for 45 minutes.
6. You can serve with 2 tbsp. E.D. Smith no sugar added syrup which will be an additional 1 POINTS.

Zucchini and Corn Frittata

Servings Per Recipe: 6, POINTS: 2
Cooking Time: minutes

Ingredients:
- 2-oz sharp cheddar cheese, shredded
- ¼ tbsp. dried chives
- ¼ tsp black pepper
- ¾ tsp salt
- 1/3 cup 2% plain Greek yogurt
- 8 large eggs
- 1 cup thin sliced zucchini
- 1 tbsp. light butter
- 1 medium ear of fresh corn

Directions:
1. Shuck the corn and place in a bowl.
2. Lightly grease with cooking spray an oven-proof skillet and preheat oven to 350°F.
3. Place skillet on medium high fire and melt butter.
4. Sauté zucchini and corn kernels for 8 minutes. Season with pepper and salt,
5. Meanwhile, in a large bowl, whisk well eggs. Stir in cheese, basil, chives, black pepper, salt, and yogurt. Mix well.
6. Once corn and zucchini are done cooking, pour them into bowl of egg mixture and mix well.
7. Then pour egg mixture back into oven-proof skillet and lower fire to medium and let it cook for 7 minutes. Transfer skillet to oven and continue cooking for 16 minutes.
8. Turn off oven and let frittata continue cooking for another 5 minutes.
9. Remove from oven, serve and enjoy.

Baked Veggie-Egg Italian Style

Servings Per Recipe: 4, POINTS: 5
Cooking Time: 60 minutes

Ingredients:

- ¼ cup grated fat-free parmesan cheese
- 4 large eggs
- ¼ tsp black pepper
- ½ tsp salt
- ½ tsp dried basil
- 2 large garlic cloves, minced
- 1 onion, halved lengthwise, sliced
- 1 zucchini, quartered lengthwise and cut crosswise into ¾-inch chunks
- 1-lb plum tomatoes, cut into 1-inch chunks

Directions:

1. Lightly grease a shallow roasting pan and preheat oven to 400°F.
2. Place onion, zucchini, bell pepper, and tomatoes in pan. Season with pepper, salt, basil, and garlic. Toss well to coat. Pop in the oven and roast for 30 minutes or until veggies are tender.
3. After roasting, lightly grease 4 ramekins or single-serve oven proof bowls with cooking spray.
4. Evenly divide roasted vegetables in the 4 bowls and make a well in the middle.
5. Break an egg in the middle of the veggies and repeat for remaining ramekins.

6. Evenly sprinkle with cheese and bake for 23 minutes or until eggs are just set.
7. Serve and enjoy.

Ham & Apricot Dijon Glaze

5 Free Style Smart Points 145 calories
TOTAL TIME: 5 hours
INGREDIENTS:
- 1 (6 to 7 pound) Hickory smoked fully cooked spiral cut ham
- 5 tbsp. apricot preserves
- 2 tablespoons Dijon mustard

DIRECTIONS:
1. Make the glaze: Whisk 4 tablespoons of preserves and mustard together.
2. Place the ham in a 6-quart or larger slow cooker, making sure you can put the lid on. You may have to turn the ham on its side if your ham is too large.
3. Brush the glaze over the ham. Cover and cook on the LOW setting for 4 to 5 hours. Brush the remaining tablespoon of preserves over the ham the 30 minutes.

NUTRITION INFORMATION
Yield: 16, Serving Size: 3 ounces
- Amount Per Serving:

Smart Points: 5, Calories: 145, Total Fat: 7g, Saturated Fat: 1.5g, Sodium: 851mg, Carbohydrates: 12g, Fiber: 0g, Sugar: 11g, Protein: 15g

Yummy Cheeseburger Soup

Cooking time: 2 hours, Serves: 4, POINTS: 7
Ingredients:
1 medium onion (chopped),
1 clove garlic (minced),
1 small stalk celery (chopped),
½ pound 93% lean ground beef,
½ cup low fat evaporated milk,
1 ½ cups chicken broth (divided),
4 ounces low fat Velveeta cheese (cubed),
Salt to taste,
Pepper to taste,
¼ teaspoon paprika to taste,
1 tablespoon all-purpose flour,
A dozen tortilla chips (crumbled)
And cooking spray

INSTRUCTIONS:
1) Place a skillet over medium heat. Spray with cooking spray.
2) Add onion, garlic, and celery and sauté until translucent. Spray the inside of the slow cooker with cooking spray. Transfer the sautéed onions into it.
3) Place the skillet back on heat and add beef. Cook until the beef is brown. Break it simultaneously as it cooks. Transfer into the slow cooker.
4) Mix in bowl flour and a little broth and add it to the skillet.
5) Place the skillet back on heat. Insert the remaining broth and always stir until thick. Scrape any brown bits that were stuck to the bottom of the skillet.
6) Transfer into the slow cooker. Add cheese, salt, pepper and evaporated milk and stir.
7) Cover and set on 'Low' for 2 hours. Ladle into soup bowls. Top with tortilla chips and serve.

Heavenly Pancakes

Ingredients:
1 tsp. sweetener, artificial
1 beaten egg white
½ Tbsp. cinnamon
½ Tbsp. baking powder
½ c. buttermilk
¾ c. whole wheat flour
1/3 c. unsweetened applesauce

Directions:
1. Combine together the egg, sweetener, cinnamon, baking powder, buttermilk, flour, and applesauce inside a bowl until there are no more lumps. Add in a bit of water to help the consistency if it is too thick.
2. Spray a bit of cooking spray on the skillet and let it heat up. When the skillet is ready, add a bit of the batter to the skillet and spread it out a bit.
3. Let these pancakes cook for a few minutes to allow the bubbles to start forming.
4. At this time, flip over the pancake and let it cook for an additional minute. Take off the heat when done and then repeat the steps with the rest of the batter until done.

Freestyle Lunch Recipes

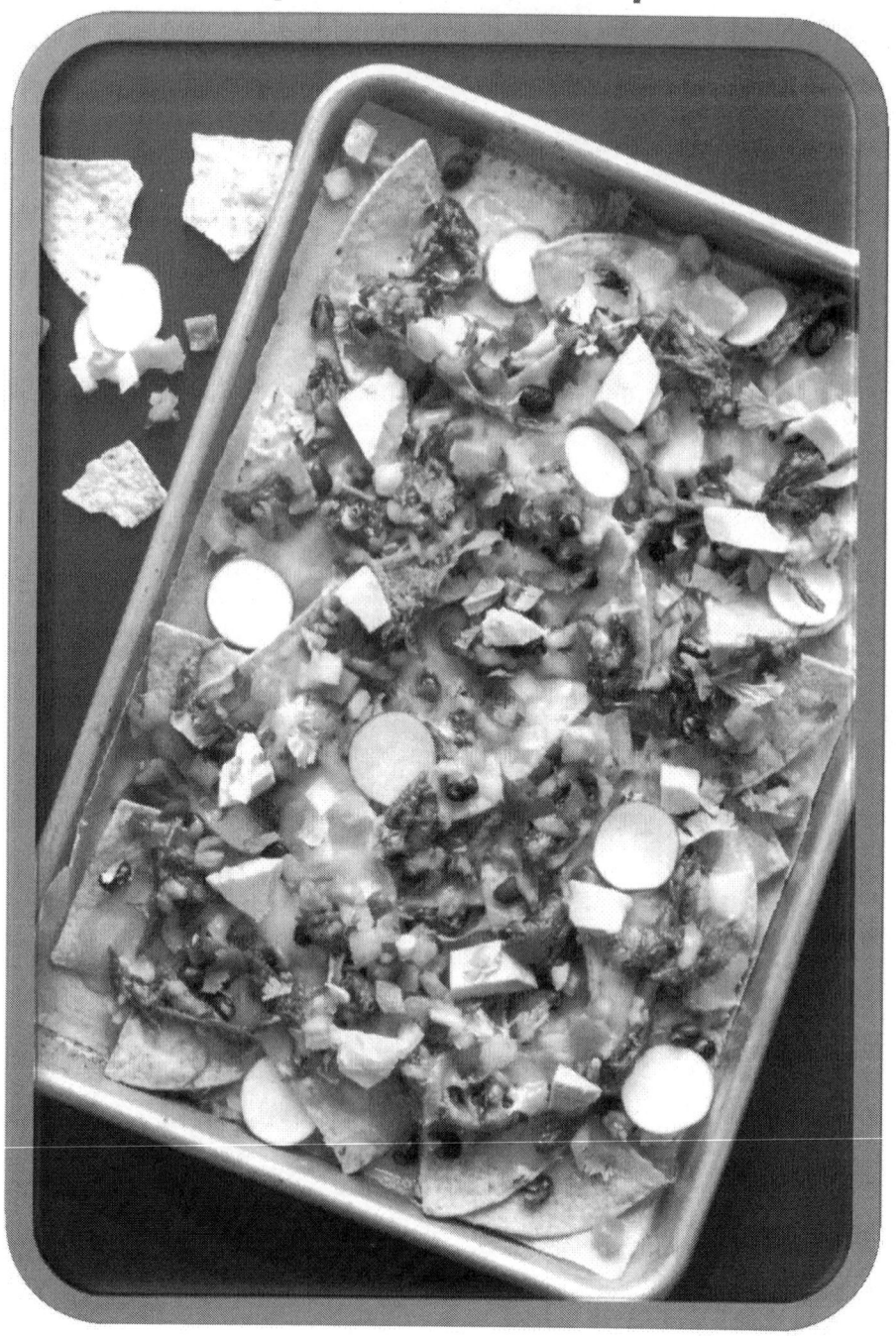

Grilled Turkey Kebabs

Servings Per Recipe: 4, POINTS: 0
Cooking Time: 10 minutes
Ingredients:
- 1 ½ pounds lean ground turkey
- 1 egg, beaten
- ½ cup minced onion
- 2 cloves of garlic, minced
- ¼ cup fresh parsley, chopped
- ½ tsp cumin
- ½ tsp garlic powder
- ½ tsp paprika
- ¼ tsp coriander
- Salt and pepper to taste

Directions:
1. Place all Ingredients: in a large mixing bowl until well combined.
2. Press the meat mixture around wooden skewers to form kebabs. Allow to set in the fridge for 30 minutes.
3. Heat the grill to high.
4. Grill the turkey kebabs for 5 minutes on each side.

Hawaiian Chicken Kebab

Servings Per Recipe: 8, POINTS: 1
Cooking Time: 12 minutes
Ingredients:
- 1-pound skinless chicken breasts, cut into 2-inch chunks
- ½ cup orange juice, freshly squeezed
- ¼ cup soy sauce
- 1 tsp garlic powder
- 1 tsp onion powder
- 1 tsp black pepper

- 1 tsp salt
- ½ tsp ginger
- ½ yellow bell pepper, seeded and cubed
- ½ red bell pepper, seeded and cubed
- ½ red onion, cut into wedges
- 1 ½ cups sliced pineapple, raw

Directions:
1. In a mixing bowl, combine the chicken in orange juice, soy sauce, garlic powder, onion powder, black pepper, salt and ginger. Marinate for 2 hours inside the fridge.
2. Slide the bell pepper, onions, and pineapple, and chicken onto the skewers alternating the meat and vegetables.
3. Heat the grill to high and cook over medium flame for 6 minutes on each side or until the meat is cooked through.

Cilantro Lime Chicken Kabobs

Servings Per Recipe: 8, POINTS: 2
Cooking Time: 10 minutes

Ingredients:
- ¼ cup cilantro, chopped
- 2 lime fruit, juiced
- 2 tbsp. olive oil
- 2 cloves of garlic, minced
- 1 tsp salt
- ½ tsp cumin
- ½ tsp paprika
- ½ tsp black pepper
- 1 ½ pounds skinless and boneless chicken breasts, chopped roughly
- 1 onion, cubed
- 2 bell peppers, cubed

Directions:

1. Place the cilantro, lime juice, olive oil, garlic, salt, cumin, paprika, and black pepper in a food processor. Pulse until smooth.
2. Place in a mixing bowl and add the chicken breasts. Allow to marinate for 2 hours in the fridge.
3. Thread the chicken, onion, and bell peppers into skewers.
4. Heat the grill to medium and cook for 5 minutes on each side.

Potato-Crusted Butter and Herb Tilapia

Servings Per Recipe: 4, POINTS: 3
Cooking Time: 12 minutes

Ingredients:
- 3 tbsp. light mayonnaise
- ½ tsp pickle relish
- ½ tsp lemon juice, freshly squeezed
- ½ tsp ground mustard
- 2 tbsp. green onions, chopped
- 4 3-ounce tilapia fillet
- ½ cup potato flakes, organic
- Salt and pepper to taste
- ½ cup butter, melted

Directions:
1. Preheat the oven to 450°F.
2. In a mixing bowl, combine the mayonnaise, pickle relish, lemon juice, mustard, and green onions.
3. Coat the tilapia fish with the mayonnaise mixture and then dredge on the potato flakes.
4. Press the potato flakes into the tilapia and sprinkle with salt and pepper to taste.
5. Place on a baking sheet and bake for 12 minutes.
6. Halfway through the cooking time, brush with butter.

Lemon Garlic Chicken and Asparagus

Servings Per Recipe: 4, POINTS: 2
Cooking Time: 19 minutes

Ingredients:
- 2 tbsp. flour
- 1 tsp garlic powder
- ½ tsp pepper
- ½ tsp salt
- 1 lemon, zest and juice
- 1 ½ pounds skinless chicken breast tenderloins, bones removed
- 1 tbsp. olive oil
- 2 cups asparagus, chopped
- 2 cloves of garlic, minced
- ½ cup chicken broth, low sodium
- 1 tbsp. white wine vinegar

Directions:
1. In a mixing bowl, combine the flour, garlic powder, pepper, salt, and lemon zest. Toss the chicken until all pieces are coated with the flour mixture.
2. Heat skillet over medium high heat and pour oil.
3. Add the coated chicken and cook on each side for 3 minutes until lightly golden.
4. Add the asparagus and garlic and cook for 3 minutes.
5. Add the chicken broth, white wine vinegar, and lemon juice. Season with more salt and pepper.
6. Close the id and simmer for 10 minutes on low heat.

Delicious Pressure Cooker Texas Red Chili

Ready in 1 hour, 6 servings, 6 Points

Ingredients

- 1 tablespoon vegetable oil
- 4-5 pounds' beef chuck roast, chopped 2 inch cubes
- ½ tablespoon kosher salt
- 2 onions, diced
- 3 cloves garlic, minced
- 2 minced chipotles with sauce
- 1/2 teaspoon kosher salt
- 1 teaspoon chili powder
- ½ cup cumin
- 2 teaspoons Mexican oregano
- 1 cup coffee
- 14 ounces can of crushed tomatoes
- Salt and pepper to taste

Instructions

1. Brown the beef: Heat the oil in the cooker pot over medium-high heat for 30 seconds. Sprinkle the beef with salt and then brown in two to three batches. Brown each batch on one side, about five minutes.

2. Add in the onions and 1/2 teaspoon of kosher salt to the cooker. Fry the onions for about 5 minutes until softened while scraping with a spoon to remove any stuck bits on the bottom. Add the garlic cloves and chipotle and then fry for one minute. Add the chili powder, oregano and cumin. Allow to cook for one minute and then stir the spices into the onions.
3. Pour the beef and any juices into the cooker, and then add the crushed tomatoes. Stir until the beef is completely coated in tomatoes and spices.
4. Shut the cooker tightly, bring the high heat and maximum pressure. Cook for 25 minutes and then release pressure naturally, about 15 minutes and then remove the lid.
5. Add salt to reduce chili bitterness. Serve the chili straight up.

Nutrition information
Calories: 225, Carbs: 7g, Fats: 16g, Proteins: 14g

Tasty Turkey Meatball & Veggie

Makes 8 servings.
One serving is 1-1/2 cups soup.
One serving is 5 FreeStyle WW SP.

INGREDIENTS
- Cooking spray
- 1 onion, chopped
- 3-4 carrots, sliced or chopped
- 1 cup green beans, cut

- 2 minced garlic cloves
- 1 (24 ounce) package Jennie-O Italian style turkey meatballs
- 2 (14.5 ounce) cans beef or vegetable broth
- 2 (14.5 ounce) diced or Italian stewed tomatoes
- 1-1/2 cups frozen corn
- 1 teaspoon oregano
- 1 teaspoon parsley
- ½ teaspoon basil

INSTRUCTIONS
1. Spray large saucepan or instant pot with cooking spray.
2. Add onions, carrots, green beans and garlic and cook over medium heat 2-3 minutes.
3. Mix in remaining ingredients.
4. If cooking on a stovetop, cover and cook over medium-low heat for 20 minutes, or until meatballs are heated through.
5. Serve warm.
6. Refrigerate or freeze leftovers.

Nutrition Information
- Calories: 285
- Fat: 13 g
- Saturated fat: 4 g
- Carbohydrates: 21 g
- Sugar: 9 g
- Sodium: 1126 mg
- Fiber: 3 g
- Protein: 19 g

GreekStyle Chickpea Salad

Nutrition Information
- Serves: 8 servings
- Serving size: ½ cup
- Calories: 192
- Fat: 4 g
- Saturated fat: 1 g
- Carbohydrates: 32 g
- Sugar: 6 g
- Fiber: 8 g
- Protein: 10 g

0 WW Freestyle SP per serving.

INGREDIENTS
- 2 (15 ounce) cans chickpea, drained and rinsed
- 1 small tomato, chopped
- ¼ cup finely chopped red onion
- ½ teaspoon sugar
- ¼ cup reduced fat crumbled feta cheese
- ½ tablespoon lemon juice
- ½ tablespoon red wine vinegar
- 1 tablespoon plain nonfat Greek Yogurt
- 2 cloves garlic, minced
- ¼ teaspoon salt
- ¼ teaspoon pepper
- 1-2 tablespoons cilantro

INSTRUCTIONS
1. Drain and rinse the chickpeas and place in a medium bowl.
2. Toss in the rest of the ingredients until chickpeas are evenly coated and all of the ingredients are mixed well.
3. Serve immediately and refrigerate any leftovers.

Tasty Freestyle Buffalo Wing Hummus

Yield: 8 (1/4 CUP) SERVINGS
INGREDIENTS:
- 1 ½ cups canned chickpeas, drained and rinsed (reserve ¼ cup of the liquid from the can)
- 2 cloves garlic
- 2 tablespoons tahini
- 2 tablespoons fresh lemon juice
- ¾ teaspoon paprika
- 1 tablespoon barbecue sauce
- 1 ½ tablespoons Frank's Red Hot (or similar cayenne pepper sauce)
- 1 ½ teaspoons white vinegar
- ¾ teaspoon salt

DIRECTIONS:
1. Combine all ingredients including the ¼ reserved liquid from the can of chickpeas into a food processor or blender. Puree ingredients until smooth. Serve.

NUTRITION INFORMATION:
72 calories, 12 g carbs, 1 g sugars, 2 g fat, 0 g saturated fat, 3 g protein, 2 g fiber

Yummy Mediterranean Bean Salad

COOKING TIME: 30 m, SERVES: 3, POINTS: 4
INGREDIENTS:
7.5 ounces canned black beans(drained, rinsed),
7.5 ounces canned garbanzo beans(drained, rinsed),
1 clove garlic(minced),

2 tablespoons fresh mint(chopped),
2 tablespoons fresh parsley(chopped),
½ cup grape tomatoes(chopped),
¼ cup red onion(chopped),
Juice of ½ lemon,
2 teaspoons olive oil,
Freshly ground pepper to taste and Kosher salt to taste

INSTRUCTIONS:

1) Add olive oil and lemon juice to a small bowl and whisk until emulsified. Add all the remaining ingredients of the salad into a bowl and mix.

2) Pour dressing over it. Toss well and set aside for 30 minutes at room temperature.

Toss well and serve

Heavenly Apple Muffin

Ingredients:
½ c. milk
2 Tbsp. vegetable oil
½ tsp. salt
½ tsp. cinnamon
1 ½ tsp. baking powder
1 c. oats
½ tsp. baking soda
2/3 c. brown sugar
2 c. shredded apple
1 ½ c. flour, all purpose

Directions:

1. Turn on the oven and let it heat up to 375 degrees. In the meantime, take out a muffin pan and grease it up.

2. Take out a bowl and combine together the milk, cinnamon, vegetable oil, baking soda, salt, brown sugar, baking powder, flour, and oats.
3. When this is all combined, pour the batter inside the muffin tin and then place into the oven.
4. Allow these to bake for 18 minutes or until they are all done. Give them some time to cool down before serving.

Sweet and Sour Meatballs

Servings Per Recipe: 6, POINTS:1
Cooking Time: 20 minutes
Ingredients:
- 1-pound ground skinless turkey breasts
- ½ tsp salt
- 1 tsp black pepper
- 1 tsp onion powder
- 1 tsp garlic powder
- 1 tsp paprika
- 1 tsp cumin
- ¼ cup teriyaki sauce
- ¼ cup BBQ sauce, sugar-free
- 1/3 cup apple cider vinegar
- 1 tbsp brown sugar

Directions:
1. In a mixing bowl, mix together the first 7 ingredients. Mix until well-combined.
2. In another bowl, mix the remaining Ingredients: to create the sauce.
3. Roll the meat mixture into 12 small balls.
4. Place the meatballs in a baking sheet lined with parchment paper.
5. Place inside a 375ºF preheated oven and bake for 10 minutes.

6. Turn the meatballs and cook for an additional 10 minutes.
7. Remove from the oven and toss in a bowl with the sauce.

One Pan Shrimp Fajitas

Servings Per Recipe: 4, POINTS: 1
Cooking Time: 8 minutes

Ingredients:
- 1 tsp chili powder
- ½ tsp paprika
- ½ tsp cumin
- ½ tsp garlic powder
- ¼ tsp oregano
- ¼ tsp salt
- ¼ tsp black pepper
- 1 ½ pounds shrimps, shelled and deveined
- 2 bell peppers, sliced thinly
- 1 onion, sliced thinly
- 1 jalapeno pepper, sliced
- 2 cloves of garlic, minced
- 1 tbsp olive oil

Directions:
1. Preheat the oven to 450°F.
2. In a mixing bowl, mix together the chili powder, paprika, cumin, garlic powder, and oregano. Season with salt and pepper to taste. This will be the fajita seasoning.
3. Place the rest of the Ingredients: in a large mixing bowl and toss in the fajita seasoning.
4. Toss to coat.
5. Place on a baking sheet and spread out the shrimps.
6. Bake for 8 minutes.
7. Turn the shrimps halfway during the cooking time.

Spaghetti Squash with Shrimps

Servings Per Recipe: 4, POINTS: 1
Cooking Time: 15 minutes

Ingredients:
- 1 spaghetti squash, large and seeded
- 1-pound asparagus, chopped
- 1 tsp olive oil
- 3 cloves of garlic, minced
- ½ cup onion, diced
- ¼ cup chicken broth, low sodium
- 1-pound shrimp, cooked and shelled
- A dash of red pepper flakes
- 1 tbsp parsley, chopped
- Salt and pepper to taste
- 2 tbsp parmesan cheese

Directions:
1. Cook the spaghetti squash in the microwave for 7 minutes. Use a fork and scrape the squash in a bowl.
2. Place the asparagus in a microwave and cook for 3 minutes. Set aside.
3. Heat the oil in a skillet over medium flame. Stir in the garlic and onions and sauté for 2 minutes. Remove from the pan and place beside the asparagus.
4. Place the broth in the skillet and allow to simmer.
5. Add the shrimps, red pepper flakes, and parsley. Season with salt and pepper to taste.
6. Assemble by placing the squash in a plate and topping it with asparagus and sautéed garlic and onions.
7. Pour in the sauce and sprinkle with parmesan cheese.

Savory Chicken Dump Soup

3 FreeStyle Smart Points per serving (approximately 12 servings / 1 cup each)

Ingredients:

- 1 pound (approx. 3-4) raw skinless boneless chicken thighs
- 1 pkg Trader Joe's frozen Multigrain Blend with Vegetables (if you don't have a TJ's first of all bless your heart.
- Second find another frozen mix with some similar combo to this: cooked grain barley, corn, spelt [wheat], whole rice ermes variety [red], whole rice ribe variety, whole rice-venus variety [black], salt), peas, carrots, water, zucchini, vinegar, extra virgin olive oil, onion, sugar, salt, pepper and totaling no more than 17 SP for the entire bag
- 2 cups (one small package) shredded cabbage
- 1 cup (one small carton fresh or one can) sliced mushrooms any type
- 6 cups water
- 2 tsp dry Italian seasoning

Directions

This first part I prep ahead and have on hand in the freezer for easy dumping. If you are anxious to try this right away though there is no need to wait! Just plan a little extra time so your family and friends don't pass out smelling all that yumminess while they stalk you in the kitchen with empty bowls in hand.

Add all of the chicken and 1/2 the water to a tall stock pot. Bring everything to a boil for 10 minutes. Reduce to a heavy simmer (not boiling, but bubbling vigorously) and cover loosely with aluminum foil. Let simmer for approximately an hour.

Remove one thigh and test with a meat thermometer. If the internal temp is not at least 150 (you want 165 when everything is done!) return and continue simmering for 15 minute intervals until chicken is completely done. If you are making this for prep, remove from heat and allow to cool. Pull chicken apart with two forks to shred or use a hand mixer to "shred" (I haven't used the hand mixer method but I want to try it!).

Return to the broth you have just made and then transfer all to a freezer safe container. If you are using immediately return everything to the stock pot and go to the next step. With your stock and shredded chicken in the stock pot, next dump all of the remaining ingredients and stir.

Bring back up to a low boil for 10 minutes, then reduce heat and simmer for 30-45 minutes

Chicken Marsala MeatBall

5 Free Style Smart Points 248 calories
TOTAL TIME: 30 minutes
INGREDIENTS:
- 8 ounces sliced cremini mushrooms, divided
- 1 pound 93% lean ground chicken
- 1/3 cup whole wheat seasoned or gluten-free bread crumbs
- 1/4 cup grated Pecorino cheese
- 1 large egg, beaten
- 3 garlic cloves, minced
- 2 tablespoons chopped fresh parsley, plus more for garnish
- 1 teaspoon Kosher salt
- Freshly ground black pepper
- 1/2 tablespoon all-purpose flour
- 1/2 tablespoon unsalted butter
- 1/4 cup finely chopped shallots
- 3 ounces sliced shiitake mushrooms
- 1/3 cup Marsala wine
- 3/4 cup reduced sodium chicken broth

DIRECTIONS:
1. Preheat the oven to 400F.
2. Finely chop half of the Cremini mushrooms and transfer to a medium bowl with the ground chicken, breadcrumbs, Pecorino, egg, 1 clove of the minced garlic, parsley, 1 teaspoon kosher salt and black pepper, to taste.
3. Gently shape into 25 small meatballs, bake 15 to 18 minutes, until golden.
4. In a small bowl whisk the flour with the Marsala wine and broth.
5. Heat a large skillet on medium heat.
6. Add the butter, garlic and shallots and cook until soft and golden, about 2 minutes.
7. Add the mushrooms, season with 1/8 teaspoon salt and a pinch of black pepper, and cook, stirring occasionally, until golden, about 5 minutes.
8. Return the meatballs to the pot, pour the Marsala wine mixture over the meatballs, cover and cook 10 minutes.
9. Garnish with parsley.

NUTRITION INFORMATION
Yield: 5 servings, Serving Size: 5 meatballs with mushrooms
- Amount Per Serving:
- Total Fat: 4g, Saturated Fat: 4g
- Cholesterol: 121mg, Sodium: 580mg
- Carbohydrates: 13g
- Fiber: 1.5g, Sugar: 4.5g, Protein: 21g

Bruschetta Topped Balsamic Chicken

Yield: 4 SERVINGS

INGREDIENTS:
- 4 (6 oz.) raw boneless skinless chicken breasts or cutlets
- Salt and pepper, to taste
- ½ teaspoon dried oregano
- 2 teaspoons olive oil, divided

- ¾ cup balsamic vinegar
- 2 tablespoons sugar
- ¼ teaspoon salt
- 1 cup chopped cherry or grape tomatoes
- 1-2 tablespoons of sliced fresh basil
- 1 teaspoon minced garlic (or more to taste)

DIRECTIONS:
1. Pre-heat the oven to 400 degrees. Place the chicken breasts on a cutting board and if necessary, pound with a meat mallet to ensure an even thickness.
2. Sprinkle each breast with salt, pepper and oregano on each side.
3. Pour 1 ½ teaspoons of olive oil into a large skillet and bring over medium-high heat.
4. Place the breasts in the pan in a single layer and cook for 1-2 minutes on each side to lightly brown the outside of the chicken.
5. Mist a baking sheet with cooking spray and place the chicken breasts onto the sheet. Cover with aluminum foil and bake for 15 minutes.
6. While the chicken is baking, combine the balsamic vinegar, sugar and salt in a small saucepan and stir to combine. Bring to a boil over medium-high heat and then reduce the heat to medium low. Simmer for 10-15 minutes until the mixture has reduced and thickened and will coat the back of a spoon. Split the balsamic glaze into two small dishes.
7. When the chicken comes out of the oven, discard any extra liquid produced by the chicken. Use a pastry brush to brush the glaze from one of the dishes onto the chicken breasts. Place the baking sheet of chicken back in the oven, uncovered this time, for 5-10 minutes until the chicken is cooked through. Wash your pastry brush thoroughly.

8. Combine the chopped tomatoes, sliced basil, minced garlic and the remaining ½ teaspoon of olive oil in a bowl and add salt and pepper to taste. Stir to combine.
9. When the chicken breasts are done cooking, brush the second dish of balsamic glaze over the chicken breasts. Serve each breast topped with ¼ cup of the bruschetta tomato mixture.

WEIGHT WATCHERS FREESTYLE SMARTPOINTS:
4 per serving (SP calculated using the recipe builder on weightwatchers.com), a serving had 7 SP on the previous program

NUTRITION INFORMATION:
293 calories, 18 g carbs, 17 g sugars, 7 g fat, 1 g saturated fat, 39 g protein, 1 g fiber .

Scrumptious Pork chops and cabbage

Ready in 20 minutes, 4 servings, 10 Points
Ingredients
- 4 pork chops, thick cut
- 1-2 teaspoon of fennel seeds
- ½ tablespoon salt
- 1 teaspoon pepper
- 1 small head of cabbage
- ¾ cup meat stock
- 1 tablespoon vegetable oil
- 2 teaspoons flour

Instructions
1. Sprinkle the pork chops with fennel, pepper and salt.
2. Slicing the cabbage into half, and then into thick ¾ inch slices then set aside.
3. Heat oil to the pre-heated pressure cooker over medium-high heat and brown all the chops and then set aside. Afterwards, add in the cabbage slices to the empty pressure cooker.
4. Arrange the pork chops on top of the cabbage brown-side up. Add in any juice from the chops.

5. Cover the cooker with lid and bring pressure to high heat and pressure. Turn up the heat high and then lower to maintain pressure. Cook for the next 6-8 minutes at high pressure.
6. Afterwards, open the cooker gently by slowly releasing the pressure.
7. Extract the cabbage and pork chops onto a serving platter. Bring the remaining juices in the pressure cooker to boil and then whisk-in the flour.
8. Pour the thickened sauce on the cabbage and pork chops platter and then serve.

Nutrition information
Calories: 366, Carbs: 22g, Fats: 22g, Proteins: 20g

Irresistible Freestyle White Chicken Chili

Yield: 8 (1 CUP) SERVINGS
INGREDIENTS:
- 1 tablespoon Canola oil
- 2 cups yellow onion, chopped
- 2 tablespoons chili powder
- 1 tablespoon minced garlic
- 2 teaspoons ground cumin
- 1 teaspoon oregano
- 3 (15.5 oz.) cans Great Northern beans, rinsed and drained
- 4 cups reduced sodium fat free chicken broth
- 3 cups chopped or shredded cooked skinless chicken breast
- 1 (14.5 oz.) can diced tomatoes
- 1/3 cup chopped fresh cilantro
- 2 tablespoon fresh lime juice
- ½ teaspoon salt
- ½ teaspoon pepper

DIRECTIONS:
1. Bring oil to medium heat in a large pot or Dutch oven. Add the onions and sauté for 5-8 minutes or until tender.

2. Add the chili powder, garlic and cumin and stir to coat the onions. Cook for 2 more minutes. Add the oregano and beans, stir and cook for 30 more seconds.
3. Add the broth and reduce the heat to medium-low. Simmer for 20 minutes, stirring occasionally.
4. Remove 2 cups of the bean/broth mixture into a blender (or container for an immersion blender) and process until smooth.
5. Return pureed mixture to the pot. Add the chicken and tomatoes and cook over medium-low for another 30 minutes, stirring occasionally.
6. Add the cilantro, lime juice, salt & pepper and stir to combine before serving.

NUTRITION INFORMATION PER 1 CUP SERVING:
291 calories, 36 g carbs, 4 g sugars, 4 g fat, 1 g saturated fat, 27 g protein, 12 g fiber

Watermelon, Jicama, & Cucumber Salad

COOKING TIME: 0m, SERVES: 3 , POINTS: 3

INGREDIENTS:
1 tablespoon olive oil,
Juice of ½ lime,
Freshly ground black pepper to taste,
Kosher salt to taste,
1 teaspoon raw honey,
1 cup jicama peeled(cubed),
1 cup watermelon(deseeded, cubed),
1 small red onion (thinly sliced),
1 medium cucumber(peeled, deseeded, cubed),
1 tablespoon fresh mint (chopped)
and 1-ounce feta cheese (crumbled or chopped into small cubes)

INSTRUCTIONS:
1) Add all the ingredients for the dressing in a small bowl and whisk until well combined.
2) Add all the salad ingredients into a bowl and toss. Pour the dressing over it and toss well.

Serve.
Delicious Mushroom and Spinach Quiche
Ingredients:
Salt
Pepper
¼ c. chopped onion
3 eggs
½ c. cottage cheese
2 tsp. garlic, minced
1 c. artichoke hearts, chopped
½ tsp. olive oil
10 oz. spinach
1 c. mushrooms, sliced
Directions:
1. Turn on the oven and let it heat up to 350 degrees. While that is heating up, take out a pan and cook together the olive oil, mushrooms, onions, and garlic.
2. When those are ready, add in the spinach and let it cook for a bit. After a few minutes, add in the rest of the ingredients and season with some pepper and salt.
3. Place this into a prepared pie dish and let it bake for 45 minutes before serving.

Salmon with Garlic Zucchini Noodles
Servings Per Recipe: 4, POINTS: 2
Cooking Time: 13 minutes
Ingredients:
- 2 tsps smoked paprika
- ½ tsp salt
- ½ tsp garlic powder
- ¼ tsp pepper
- ¼ tsp dried oregano
- 1/8 tsp chili powder

- 1 ½ pounds wild salmon fillets, skin removed
- 2 tbsps olive oil
- 2 cloves of garlic, minced
- 2 zucchinis, cut into long strips
- 1 cup cherry tomatoes
- 1 lemon, cut into wedges

Directions:
1. Create the spice rub by mixing the first 6 Ingredients: in a bowl.
2. Rub the mixture onto the salmon fillets.
3. Heat half of the oil in a skillet over medium flame and cook the salmon for 4 minutes per side. Set aside.
4. Add the remaining oil and sauté the garlic until fragrant.
5. Stir in the zucchini and tomatoes and cook for another 5 minutes.
6. Serve the vegetables with the salmon and add lemon wedges on top.

Easy Turkey Chili

Servings Per Recipe: 4, POINTS:1
Cooking Time: 30 minutes

Ingredients:
- ½ tbsp olive oil
- 1 onion, chopped
- 2 cloves of garlic, minced
- 1 red pepper, chopped
- ½ cup celery, chopped
- 1 jalapeno pepper, seeded and diced
- 2 tbsps chipotle pepper, diced
- 1-pound lean ground turkey meat
- 1 ½ tbsps chili powder
- 1 tsp oregano
- 1 tsp ground cumin
- 1 bay leaf
- 1 cup tomatoes, diced

- ¾ cup chicken broth, low sodium
- Salt and pepper to taste
- 1 can kidney beans, rinsed and drained

Directions:
1. Heat oil in a skillet over medium flame.
2. Sauté the onion, garlic, red pepper, celery, jalapeno, and chipotle. Stir constantly for 5 minutes.
3. Stir in the turkey, chili powder, oregano, and ground cumin and cook for another 5 minutes.
4. Add the rest of the ingredients.
5. Allow to simmer for 20 minutes.

Tasty Whole Chicken in an Instant Pot

Ready in 55 minutes, 6 servings, 8 Points

Ingredients
- 1 whole chicken
- Any preferred seasonings
- 1 cup water
- 1 tablespoon coconut oil

Directions
1. Put a cup of water into the Instant Pot and add in the steam rack.
2. Heat the oil in a large skillet.
3. Coat the chicken with seasonings and then place in the oil and allow to brown for at least one minute on each side and then withdraw from heat.
4. Transfer the chicken to the Instant Pot on the steam rack.
5. Tight lid the Instant Pot and set to Chicken on high pressure. Adjust the time. Allow chicken to cook for not more than 30 minutes and the release steam naturally for 15 minutes. You can as well save the bones and make broth instead of throwing them.

Nutrition information
Calories: 339, Carbohydrates: 1g, Fats: 19g
Proteins: 38g

Freestyle Dinner Recipes

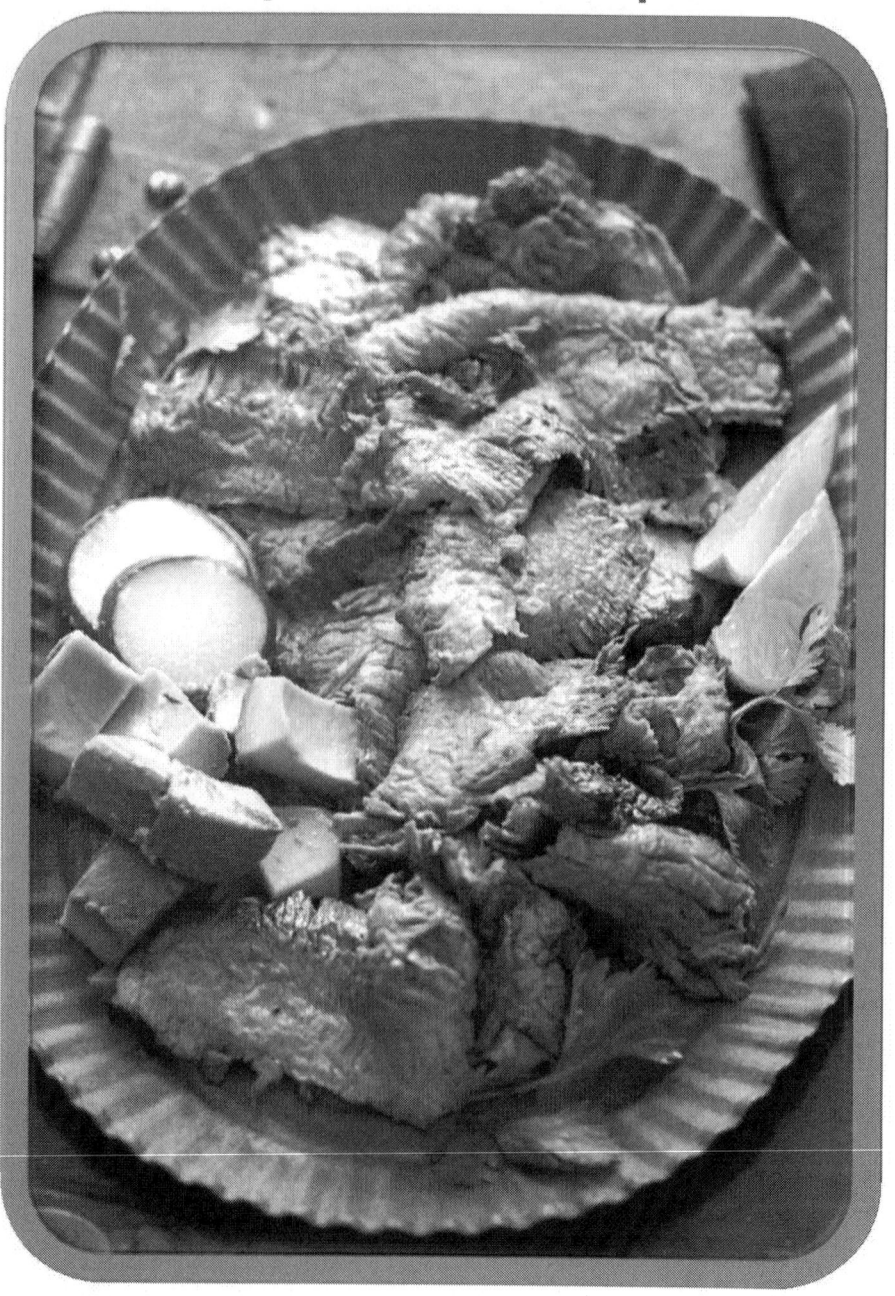

Delicious Pressure Cooker Red Beans and Rice

Ready in 8 hrs. 45 minutes,
8 servings
10 Points
Ingredients
- Beans and soaking
- Pound beans, well sorted and rinsed
- 1 tablespoon kosher salt
- 2 quarts' water
- Aromatics
- 2 teaspoon vegetable oil
- 1 pound smoked sausage quartered into 1/4 inch wedges
- 1 large onion, minced
- 1 stalk celery, minced
- 1 green bell pepper, seeded and minced
- 4 cloves garlic, thinly sliced
- 1 teaspoon fresh thyme leaves
- 1 teaspoon salt
- 2 bay leaves
- 1 teaspoon salt
- 5 cups water
- salt and pepper
- For serving
- Cooked long grain white rice
- Parsley minced
- Green onions, minced
- Hot sauce

Directions

1. Sort the beans, and remove broken beans, dirt and stones. Rinse and transfer into a large container add one tablespoon of salt and cover with 2 quarts' water.
2. Heat oil in the pressure cooker over medium heat until it shimmers and add the smoked sausage, garlic, onion, celery, bell pepper, thyme and sprinkle with salt. fry for 8 minutes until the onions and sausage turn brown around the edges.
3. Drain the beans and rinse. Pour them into the pressure cooker, add bay leaves and 1 teaspoon of salt, and then stir in the water. Tightly lid the pressure cooker and allow to cook at high pressure for the next 15 minutes. Release pressure naturally for about 20 minutes. Carefully remove the lid.
4. Discard the bay leaves. Scoop out 2 cups of the beans and the liquid, puree, and pour back into the pot. Simmer for another fifteen minutes. Taste to check seasoning and serve.

Nutrition information
Calories: 838, Carbohydrates: 140g, Fats: 20g, Proteins: 23g

Chicken Marsala Meatballs

Servings Per Recipe: 10, POINTS: 5
Cooking Time: 30 minutes

Ingredients:
- 8 ounces cremini mushrooms, chopped finely
- 1-pound lean ground chicken
- 1/3 cup whole wheat bread crumbs
- ¼ cup pecorino cheese, grated
- 1 large egg, beaten
- 2 tablespoons chopped parsley
- 3 cloves of garlic, minced
- 1 teaspoon salt
- A dash of black pepper
- ½ tablespoon all-purpose flour
- 1/3 cup Marsala wine
- ¾ cup chicken broth, low sodium
- ½ tablespoon unsalted butter
- ¼ cup shallots, chopped
- 3 ounces sliced shiitake mushrooms

Directions:
1. Preheat the oven to 400°F.
2. In a mixing bowl, combine the cremini mushrooms, chicken, bread crumbs, cheese, egg, parsley, garlic, salt, and pepper. Mix until well combined.
3. Form small balls using your hands and place in a greased baking sheet.
4. Bake for 20 minutes.

5. Meanwhile, make the sauce by combining the all-purpose flour, Marsala wine, and broth. Set aside.
6. Heat the butter in a skillet over medium flame and sauté the shallots until fragrant.
7. Stir in the mushrooms and cook for another 3 minutes.
8. Pour in the broth and allow to simmer for 5 minutes until it thickens.
9. Toss the cooked meatballs in to coat the sauce.

Simple Vegan Potato Soup

Servings Per Recipe:10, POINTS: 3
Cooking Time: 35 minutes

Ingredients:
- 1 tablespoon olive oil
- 2 leeks, sliced thinly
- 1 onion, diced
- 3 cloves of garlic, minced
- 1 carrot, diced
- 2 cups potatoes, peeled and cubed
- 4 cups vegetable broth
- 2 cups water
- 2 cups rice milk
- 2 tablespoons vegan butter
- ½ cup instant potato flakes, organic
- 2 teaspoons salt
- 2 teaspoons black pepper
- 1 teaspoon onion powder
- 1 teaspoon garlic powder
- 1 teaspoon smoked paprika

Directions:
1. In a large pot, heat the oil over medium flame and sauté the leeks, onion, garlic, and carrots for 3 minutes.
2. Add the potatoes, vegetable broth, water, and rice milk. Bring to a boil.
3. Once boiled, add the rest of the Ingredients.
4. Allow to simmer for 25 minutes.

African Sweet Potato Stew

Servings Per Recipe: 6, POINTS: 4
Cooking Time: 8 hours

Ingredients:
- 1 ¼ pounds sweet potatoes, peeled and cubed
- 2 cups diced tomatoes
- 1 can red beans, drained and rinsed
- 4 cups vegetable broth
- ½ cup water
- 1 onion, chopped
- 1 bell pepper, chopped
- 2 cloves of garlic, minced
- 1 teaspoon grated fresh ginger
- ½ teaspoon salt
- 1 teaspoon cumin powder
- ¼ teaspoon black pepper
- 3 tablespoons creamy peanut butter

Directions:
1. Place all the Ingredients: except for the peanut butter in the slow cooker.

2. Cover the lid and cook on low for 8 hours.
3. An hour before the cooking time, spoon ½ cup of the stew liquid into a bowl and dilute the peanut butter into it.
4. Stir the peanut butter mixture into the stew.
5. Close the lid and continue cooking until done.

Slow Cooker Chicken and Tomato Orzo

Servings Per Recipe: 8, POINTS: 4
Cooking Time: 6 hours

Ingredients:
- 1-pound boneless chicken breasts
- 1 tablespoon olive oil
- 2 tablespoons garlic salt
- 1 tablespoon black pepper
- 2 cups chicken broth
- 8-ounce package orzo
- 2 tablespoons minced garlic
- 1 pack tomatoes, halved
- 4 tablespoons parmesan cheese, grated

Directions:
1. Place the chicken breasts, olive oil, garlic salt, pepper, and broth in a slow cooker.
2. Close the lid and cook on low for 6 hours.
3. An hour before the cooking time ends, Add the orzo, garlic, and tomatoes. Stir to combine.
4. Continue cooking.
5. Serve parmesan cheese last.

Tasty Turkey Meatball & Veggie Soup

Nutrition Information
Calories: 285, Fat: 13 g, Saturated fat: 4 g
Trans fat: 0 g, Carbohydrates: 21 g, Sugar: 9 g
Sodium: 1126 mg, Fiber: 3 g, Protein: 19 g
Makes 8 servings.
One serving is 1-1/2 cups soup.
One serving is 5 FreeStyle WW SP.

INGREDIENTS
- Cooking spray
- 1 onion, chopped
- 3-4 carrots, sliced or chopped
- 1 cup green beans, cut
- 2 minced garlic cloves
- 1 (24 ounce) package Jennie-O Italian style turkey meatballs
- 2 (14.5 ounce) cans beef or vegetable broth
- 2 (14.5 ounce) diced or Italian stewed tomatoes
- 1-1/2 cups frozen corn
- 1 teaspoon oregano
- 1 teaspoon parsley
- ½ teaspoon basil

INSTRUCTIONS
1. Spray large saucepan or instant pot with cooking spray.
2. Add onions, carrots, green beans and garlic and cook over medium heat 2-3 minutes.
3. Mix in remaining ingredients.

4. If cooking on a stovetop, cover and cook over medium-low heat for 20 minutes, or until meatballs are heated through.

Sticky Buffalo Chicken Tenders

Prep time: 10 mins
Cook time: 15 mins
Total time: 25 mins

Ingredients
- 1 pound boneless skinless chicken breasts, pounded to ½" thickness
- ¼ cup flour
- 3 eggs
- 1 cup Italian Seasoned Panko breadcrumbs
- ½ cup brown sugar
- ⅓ cup Frank's Red Hot Sauce
- ½ teaspoon Garlic Powder
- 3 tablespoons water

Instructions
1. Preheat oven to 425 degrees and spray a baking sheet with non-stick cooking spray or line with silicone baking mats.
2. Cut boneless skinless chicken breasts into strips or chunks (we find chunks hold coating better).
3. Add the chicken into a large Ziploc bag that contains just the flour. Shake to coat.
4. Place Panko breadcrumbs into a shallow bowl. In another shallow bowl, whisk eggs until combined well.
5. Dip flour coated chicken into eggs, then into Panko breadcrumbs to coat.

6. Place coated chicken on the prepared baking sheet. Spray tops with non-stick cooking spray.
7. Bake for 15 minutes for nuggets or 20 minutes for strips or until chicken is browned and cooked through.
8. While chicken is in the oven, you will make your sauce mixture.
9. In a medium saucepan, bring the brown sugar, garlic powder, water and Frank's red hot sauce to a boil. Remove from heat and stir well.
10. When chicken is cooked through, remove from the oven and toss with sauce. This will just coat the chicken.

Makes 6 Servings
7 PointsPlus per Serving
8 SmartPoints per Serving on Beyond the Scale
5 SmartPoints per Serving on FreeStyle or Flex Plan

Slow Cook Chicken Cacciatore

INGREDIENTS:
- 8 bone-in, skinless chicken thighs
- 3/4 teaspoon kosher salt
- freshly ground black pepper
- cooking spray
- 5 garlic cloves, finely chopped
- 1/2 large onion, chopped
- 1 28-ounce can crushed tomatoes
- 1/2 medium red bell pepper, chopped
- 1/2 medium green bell pepper, chopped
- 4 ounce sliced shiitake mushrooms
- 1 sprig of fresh thyme

- 1 sprig of fresh oregano
- 1 bay leaf
- 1 tablespoon chopped fresh parsley (I omitted this)
- freshly grated Parmesan cheese, for serving (optional)

DIRECTIONS:
1. Season the chicken with salt and pepper to taste. Heat a large nonstick skillet over medium-high heat.
2. Coat with cooking spray, add the chicken, and cook until browned- 2 to 3 minutes per side. Transfer to your slow cooker.
3. Reduce the heat under the skillet to medium and coat with more cooking spray. Add the garlic and onion and cook, stirring, until soft- 3 to 4 minutes.
4. Transfer to the slow cooker and add the tomatoes, bell peppers, mushrooms, thyme, oregano and bay leaf. Stir to combine.
5. Cover and cook on high for 4 hours or on low for 8 hours.
6. Discard the bay leaf and transfer the chicken to a large plate. Pull the chicken meat from the bones (discard the bones), shred the meat, and return it to the sauce.
7. Stir in the parsley (if using). If desired, serve topped with Parmesan cheese.

Nutritional information per serving: Calories: 220, Fat: 6g, Sat Fat: 1.5g, Cholesterol: 123mg, Sodium: 319mg, Carbohydrates: 10g, Fiber: 2g, Sugar: 6g, Protein: 31g

Weight Watchers POINTS: Freestyle SmartPoints: 0 (but only if you use chicken breast instead of thighs), Original SmartPoints: 3, PointsPlus: 5, Old Program: 5

Garlic Roasted Garbanzo Beans

Prep time: 5 mins, Cook time: 45 mins
Total time: 50 mins

Ingredients
- 1 can garbanzo beans (chickpeas)
- 1 tablespoon olive oil
- 1 teaspoon salt
- 1 teaspoon garlic powder
- ½ teaspoon paprika

Instructions
1. Preheat oven to 375° Fahrenheit.
2. Line a baking sheet with a silicone baking mat or parchment paper.
3. Drain and rinse the garbanzo beans.
4. Pat garbanzo beans dry, pour into a large bowl.
5. Toss with olive oil, salt, garlic powder, and paprika until all are well coated.
6. Spread evenly over baking sheet.
7. Bake at 375° for 20 minutes. Turn chickpeas so they are evenly roasted (use a spatula to flip them or simply stir around but make sure they are in an even layer).
8. Place back in the oven at 375° for additional 25 minutes.
9. Allow the roasted garbanzo beans to cool before storing in an airtight container for snacking.

Makes approximately 3 servings
5 SmartPoints per 1/2 cup on Beyond the Scale, FreeStyle, and Flex Plan

Sea Scallops, Arugula, & Beet Salad

COOKING TIME: 6 minutes, SERVES: 2, POINTS: 7

INGREDIENTS:
- 1 tablespoon olive oil,
- ½ tablespoon red wine vinegar,
- 1 teaspoon shallot(minced),
- ½ tablespoon cider vinegar,
- ¾ tablespoon raw honey,
- 2.5 ounces baby arugula,
- 1 cup yellow beets(peeled, diced, cooked),
- 6 large sea scallops,
- Pepper to taste,
- Kosher salt to taste,
- 2 tablespoons goat cheese,
- crumbled,
- 4 grape tomatoes (halved),
- and Cooking spray

INSTRUCTIONS:
1) Sprinkle salt and pepper over the scallops. Place a nonstick pan over medium-high heat. Spray with cooking spray.
2) Add scallops. Do not stir and sear until golden brown in color.
3) Flip sides and cook the other side until golden brown. Do not overcook.
4) To make the dressing: Whisk together all the ingredients for the dressing and set aside.
5) Pour dressing over the arugula and toss. Divide the arugula among 2 plates.
6) Top with half the beets, half the tomato, 3 scallops and half the goat cheese over the arugula in the 2 plates.
7) Serve immediately.

Scrumptious Cheese and Ham Omelet

Ingredients:
½ c. diced ham
¼ c. Parmesan cheese
1/8 tsp. pepper
1/8 tsp. hot pepper sauce
2 Tbsp. green onion, chopped
¼ tsp. salt
2 eggs
4 egg whites

Directions:
1. For this recipe, bring out a bowl and ix together the hot sauce, salt, pepper, eggs, and onion.
2. Take out a skillet and grease it with some cooking spray before heating it up. Pour the mixture into the skillet and let it cook for 5 minutes so it has time to set.
3. Sprinkle the top with the ham and the Parmesan cheese. Fold the omelet in half and let it cook for another minute before serving.

Heavenly Beans & Vegan Nachos In the Pot

Ready in 45 minutes, 5 servings, 12 Points
Ingredients
- 2 cups of dried beans, well rinsed
- 1/2 tablespoon salt
- 5 cloves of garlic, peeled and chopped
- 1 jalapeno - seeded
- 1 diced large onion
- 1 teaspoon paprika
- ½ teaspoon chili powder
- 1 teaspoon cumin
- ½ teaspoon black pepper
- ½ cup salsa
- 4 cups of vegetable broth

Instructions

1. Add all the ingredients into the instant pot and stir well. Tightly close with the lid. Seal the steam valve. Shorten cooking time to about 30 minutes.
2. Leave for at least 10 minutes before releasing the pressure. Open the lid and stir well.
3. Blend the beans to by either mashing in the potato masher, or blending. Drain some of the water off before mashing or blending, and add it back just as you need it to thicken the beans according to preference.
4. Serve warm

Nutrition information
Calories: 613, Cars: 58.4g, Fats: 32g, Proteins: 25.4g

Freestyle Corn & Zucchini Summer Frittata

Yield: 6 SLICES
INGREDIENTS:
- 1 medium ear of fresh raw corn
- 1 tablespoon light butter (I use Land O'Lakes)
- 1 cup thin sliced zucchini
- 8 large eggs
- 1/3 cup 2% plain Greek yogurt (I used Fage)
- ¾ teaspoon salt (plus a sprinkle more for the corn & zucchini)
- ¼ teaspoon black pepper (plus a sprinkle more for the corn & zucchini)
- 1 tablespoon diced chives
- ¼ cup sliced fresh basil
- 2 oz. sharp cheddar cheese, shredded (I used Cabot Seriously Sharp)

DIRECTIONS:
1. Pre-heat your oven to 350. Shuck the corn and remove any remaining strings. Use a large sharp knife to cut off the kernels as close to the cob as you can get (I ended up with about 1 cup of kernels).

2. Melt the butter in an 8"-10" *oven-safe* nonstick deep skillet over medium-low heat. Add the corn kernels and the sliced zucchini and stir to coat.
3. Sprinkle with a bit of salt and pepper to taste. Cook, stirring regularly, for 6-8 minutes or until corn and zucchini are cooked through.
4. While the corn and zucchini are cooking, break the eggs into a large mixing bowl and whisk together until just combined.
5. Add the yogurt, salt, black pepper, chives, basil and shredded cheese and stir together until mixed.
6. When the corn and zucchini are cooked, transfer them into the bowl containing the egg mixture and stir together. Spray the skillet you used liberally with cooking spray and then pour the egg mixture into the skillet.
7. Cook on a burner set to medium heat for 5-7 minutes until the very outside edge of the frittata starts to turn opaque/look cooked.
8. Transfer the skillet into the oven and cook for 15-17 minutes until the center is set. Let cool for 5 minutes, then slice into 6 slices and serve.

NUTRITION INFORMATION PER SLICE:
167 calories, 5 g carbs, 2 g sugars, 11 g fat, 5 g saturated fat, 13 g protein, 1 g fiber

Spiralized Apple & Cabbage Slaw

COOKING TIME: 5-8 minutes, SERVES: 3, POINTS: 2
INGREDIENTS:
- 1 ½ cups red cabbage(shredded),
- 1 cup green cabbage(shredded),
- 1 small Granny Smith apple (discard stem),
- 1 tablespoon golden balsamic vinegar,
- 1 tablespoon olive oil,
- 1 teaspoon honey,

- ¾ teaspoon poppy seeds,
- Freshly ground black pepper to taste and Kosher salt to taste

INSTRUCTIONS:

1) Add olive oil, vinegar, poppy seeds, honey, salt, and pepper into a bowl and whisk well.

2) Make noodles of the apple using a spiralizer using a larger blade. Once the noodles are made, cut into smaller pieces using scissors. Place in a bowl.

3) Add cabbage, red as well as white. Pour dressing over it and fold gently until well combined.

Serve as it is or chills and serve later.

Lentil and Vegetable Stew

Servings Per Recipe: 6, POINTS:4
Cooking Time: 8 hours and 30 minutes

Ingredients:
- 2 cups butternut squash, peeled and cubed
- 2 cups carrots, chopped
- 2 cups red potatoes, chopped
- 2 cups celery, chopped
- 1 ½ cups dry lentils, soaked overnight and rinsed
- 1 onions, diced
- 4 cloves of garlic, minced
- 8 cups vegetable broth
- 2 teaspoons herb de Provence
- 1 teaspoon salt
- 1 teaspoon smoked paprika
- 2 tablespoons olive oil
- Salt and pepper to taste
- 4 cups spinach
- ½ cup parsley

Directions:
1. Place all Ingredients: in the slow cooker except for the spinach and parsley.
2. Close the lid and cook on low for8 hours.
3. Place a blender and pulse until smooth.

4. Return to the crockpot and add the spinach and parsley.
5. Cook on high for 30 minutes.

Beef Italian Soup

Servings Per Recipe: 8, POINTS:1
Cooking Time: 30 minutes

Ingredients:
- ½ teaspoon olive oil
- ½ pound lean round steak, sliced
- ½ cup chopped onions
- 1 teaspoon Italian seasoning mix
- ¼ teaspoon garlic salt
- ¼ teaspoon pepper
- 1 can diced tomatoes, low-sodium
- ½ cup chopped carrots
- 1 can white kidney beans, rinsed and drained
- 2 cans beef broth, fat-free and low-sodium
- 2 ½ cups shredded cabbage
- ¼ cup snipped parsley

Directions:
1. Heat the oil in a pot over medium flame and stir in meat and onions. Stir for 3 minutes.
2. Season with Italian seasoning mix, garlic, salt and pepper and stir for 2 minutes.
3. Stir in the tomatoes, carrots, kidney beans and broth.
4. Bring to a boil and allow to simmer for 20 minutes.
5. Add the cabbages and parsley and allow to simmer for 5 more minutes.

Greek Lemon Chicken Soup

Servings Per Recipe: 4
POINTS: 2
Cooking Time: 30 minutes

Ingredients:

- 2 cups cooked chicken, chopped
- 2 medium carrots, chopped
- ½ cup onion, chopped
- ¼ cup lemon juice
- 1 clove of garlic, minced
- 1 can cream of chicken soup, fat-free and low-sodium
- 2 cans chicken broth, fat-free
- ¼ teaspoon ground black pepper
- 2/3 cup uncooked long-grain rice
- 2 tablespoons parsley, snipped

Directions:

1. Place all Ingredients: in a pot except for the rice and parsley.
2. Season with salt and pepper to taste.
3. Bring to a boil.
4. Once the broth is boiling hot, stir in the rice.
5. Adjust the flame to medium and allow to simmer for 20 minutes until the rice is tender.
6. Garnish with parsley on top.

Turkey Vegetable Soup

Servings Per Recipe: 6, POINTS: 0
Cooking Time: 23 minutes

Ingredients:
- 1 cup chopped celery
- ½ cup onion, chopped
- 1 ½ teaspoon minced garlic
- 1 ½ pounds ground turkey breasts, skinless
- 6 cups chicken broth, fat-free and low-sodium
- 1 cup carrot, sliced
- ½ cup fresh green beans, cut into 1-inch length
- ½ cup frozen whole kernel corn
- 1 ½ teaspoons ground cumin
- 1 teaspoon chili power
- 2 bay leaves
- 1 can kidney beans, rinsed and drained
- 1 can diced tomatoes and green chilies, undrained
- 6 tablespoons Monterey Jack cheese, grated

Directions:
1. Heat a non-stick pan over medium heat and add the celery, onion, garlic, and turkey. Stir for 3 minutes.
2. Add the rest of the Ingredients: except the cheese.
3. Close the lid and bring to a boil.
4. Allow to simmer for 20 minutes.
5. Serve with cheese on top.

Sweet & Sour Turkey Meatballs

Prep time:5 m, Cook time:15 m, Total time:20 m
Serves:6

Ingredients
- 1 pound 99% Ground Turkey breast or Ground Chicken Breast
- ½ Teaspoon Salt
- 1 Teaspoon Black Pepper
- 1 Teaspoon Onion Powder
- 1 Teaspoon Garlic Powder
- 1 Teaspoon Paprika
- 1 Teaspoon Cumin
- ¼ teriyaki sauce
- ¼ Cup Sugar-Free BBQ Sauce
- ⅛ cup apple cider vinegar
- 1 tablespoon brown sugar twin

Instructions
1. In a large bowl, mix together ground meat and spices (salt, pepper, onion powder, garlic powder, paprika, and cumin). Mix until well blended.
2. In a small bowl, mix together the teriyaki sauce, BBQ sauce, apple cider vinegar, and brown sugar twin.
3. Add ¼ cup of sauce mixture to meat mixture and mix well.
4. Roll meat mixture into 1½" balls. Should make about 12 meatballs
5. Place meatballs on a lined baking sheet (we use silicone baking mats) about 1" apart
6. Bake at 375 degrees for 10 minutes. Turn meatballs, and cook for additional 10 minutes.
7. Remove from oven and toss with sauce until well coated.

WW Information:
Makes 6 servings of 3 meatballs per serving
1 SmartPoint on FreeStyle Plan or Flex Plan

Tasty BBQ Apricot Chicken

Prep time:5 m, Cook time:30 m, Total time:35 m
Serves:6

Ingredients
- 1 pound boneless skinless chicken breasts
- ½ cup sugar-free apricot jam
- ½ cup G Hughes Sugar Free BBQ Sauce
- 2 tablespoons low sodium soy sauce
- 1 teaspoon garlic powder
- 1 teaspoon onion powder
- 1 teaspoon ground ginger

Instructions
1. In a medium bowl, whisk together the jam, bbq sauce, soy sauce, and seasonings.
2. Line baking sheet with foil and place chicken breasts in even layer
3. Pour barbecue sauce over chicken making sure well covered.
4. Bake at 350 degrees for 30 minutes.
5. Remove from oven, and serve with favorite sides.

WW Information:
Makes 6 Servings (approximately 3oz each)
2 SmartPoints per serving on Freestyle or FlexPlan

Pizza Lasagna Roll-Ups

Yield:8 PIECES
INGREDIENTS:
- 8 uncooked lasagna noodles
- 15 oz. can tomato sauce
- 1 cup pizza sauce
- ½ teaspoon Italian seasoning
- 1 lb. uncooked hot Italian poultry sausage, casings removed if present (I used Wegmans patties, you can use chicken or turkey sausage)
- 2 oz. turkey pepperoni, chopped (reserve 8 slices un-chopped for topping)
- 1 (15 oz.) container fat free Ricotta cheese

- 1 (10 oz.) package frozen chopped spinach, thawed and squeezed until dry
- 1 large egg
- 2 oz. 2% shredded Mozzarella cheese

DIRECTIONS:
1. Pre-heat the oven to 350. Lightly mist a 9×13 baking dish with cooking spray and set aside.
2. Boil and salt a large pot of water and cook lasagna noodles according to package instructions. Drain and rinse with cold water. Lay noodles flat on a clean dry surface and set aside.
3. In a mixing bowl, combine the tomato sauce, pizza sauce and Italian seasoning and stir together. Set aside.
4. Place the sausage in a large skillet over medium heat and cook until browned, breaking the meat up into small pieces as it cooks. When the sausage is cooked through, add the chopped pepperoni and 1/3 cup of the tomato sauce mixture and stir to combine. Remove from heat.
5. In a mixing bowl, combine the ricotta cheese, spinach and egg and stir until well combined. Spoon 1/3 cup of the cheese mixture onto each lasagna noodle and spread across the surface leaving a little room (about ½") at the far end with no toppings. Top the cheese layer on each noodle with the meat mixture from step four, evenly dividing the meat between the noodles. Starting with one end (not the one with space at the end), roll the noodle over the filling until it becomes a complete roll. Repeat with all noodles.

6. Spoon ½ cup of the tomato sauce mixture into the prepared baking dish and spread across the bottom. Place the lasagna rolls seam down in the dish and spoon or pour the remaining sauce over top. Sprinkle the Mozzarella over the top of the rolls and place a pepperoni on each one. Cover the dish with aluminum foil and bake for 40 minutes.

WEIGHT WATCHERS FREESTYLE SMARTPOINTS:
7 per serving
NUTRITION INFORMATION:
289 calories, 31 g carbs, 9 g sugars, 8 g fat, 2 g saturated fat, 24 g protein, 4 g fiber

Delicious Crispy Apple Surprise

Ingredients:
- Ground cloves
- 3 lb. sliced apples
- ¼ c. sugar
- 1 tsp. vanilla
- ¼ tsp. nutmeg
- 3 Tbsp. butter
- 1 tsp. water
- ¼ tsp. cinnamon
- Salt
- ¼ c. brown sugar
- ½ tsp. ginger
- ½ c. and 2 Tbsp. flour
- ½ c. quick cooking oats

Directions;
1. For this recipe, turn on the oven and let it heat up to 375 degrees. Take out a baking dish and cover it with some cooking spray.
2. First we will need to make the topping. To do this, bring out a bowl and combine the oats with the cinnamon, salt, brown sugar, ginger, and ½ cup of flour.

3. Add in the butter at this time and then place it all into the pastry blender so that you get a nice crumbly mixture. Pour in some water and then press this to make clumps.
4. Now you will want to work on the filling. To do this, bring out a bowl and combine the cloves, sugar, nutmeg, and the rest of the flour. Put in the vanilla and the apples in as well and then pour everything inside a baking dish.
5. Pour your topping over the filling and then place everything into the oven. Bake this all in the oven for 60 minutes.

Tasty Pressure cooked beef ribs

Ready in 25-30 minutes, 2 servings, 2 Points
Ingredients
- 1 rack of beef back ribs
- Dry rub
- ½ cup kosher salt
- ½ cup water
- 4 ounces of applesauce, unsweetened
- 2 tablespoons coconut oil
- 1 teaspoon fish sauce

Instructions
1. Dry the beef back ribs with a paper towel and then, sprinkle with the dry rub and salt. Wrap up in foil and set aside to marinate for two hours.
2. Preheat the broiler, grab the rack from the fridge and cut to fit in the pressure cooker. Put the ribs on a wire rack in a baking sheet rimmed and foil lined.
3. Broil the ribs for 1-2 minutes each side. Add water, fish sauce applesauce and coconut oil to the pressure cooker and stir to combine, add a rack to the pot.

4. Put the ribs into the cooker and tight lid. Bring the heat to high pressure and lower to maintain high pressure. Cook for 20 minutes and release pressure naturally and quickly.
5. Withdraw the ribs and place them back on a wire rack lined with foil and rimmed baking sheet.
6. Simmer the remaining cooking liquid for 5 minutes and skim off any excess fat and adjust seasoning.
7. Coat the racks with the remaining liquid and broil them for one minute.

Nutrition information
Calories: 87, Carbs: 0g, Fats: 7g, Proteins: 4.7g

Freestyle Ham and Cheese Egg Cups

Yield: 12 EGG CUPS
INGREDIENTS:
- 9 oz. thinly sliced deli ham, divided (I used Hillshire Farm Deli Select)
- 6 large eggs
- 2 egg whites
- ¼ cup skim milk
- ¼ teaspoon salt
- 1/8 teaspoon pepper
- ½ cup chopped fresh spinach leaves
- 2 oz. shredded 2% sharp cheddar cheese, divided

DIRECTIONS:
1. Preheat the oven to 350. Lightly mist 12 cups in a muffin tin with cooking spray. Press a slice of ham into each cup of the muffin tin, arranging the edges to form a ham cup.
2. Chop up the remaining ham (my slices were about ½ ounce each so I had around 3 ounces remaining) and set aside.

3. In a mixing bowl, combine the eggs, egg whites, milk, salt and pepper and whisk together until yolks and whites are fully combined and beaten.
4. Add the reserved chopped ham, the spinach and half of the shredded cheddar and stir together to combine.
5. Spoon the egg mixture evenly into the ham cups and then top each cup with the remaining shredded cheese. Place the tin in the oven and bake for 18-20 minutes until the eggs are set.

NUTRITION INFORMATION PER EGG CUP:
82 calories, 2 g carbs, 1 g sugars, 4 g fat, 2 g saturated fat, 9 g protein, 0 g fiber

Heavenly Low Yolk Egg Salad

COOKING TIME: 5 minutes, SERVES: 4, POINTS: 5
INGREDIENTS:
8 eggs (hard boiled, peeled),
1 teaspoon Dijon mustard,
8 teaspoons light mayonnaise,
4 tablespoons green scallions or chives,
Freshly ground black pepper and Salt to taste
INSTRUCTIONS:
1) Separate the yolks from the whites. Use only 2 yolks and discard the rest. Chop the 2 yolks and all the whites and place in a bowl.
2) Add rest of the ingredients and fold gently.

Sticky Buffalo Chicken Tenders

Servings Per Recipe: 6, POINTS: 5
Cooking Time: 20 minutes

Ingredients:
- 1-pound skinless chicken breasts, pounded into ½" thickness
- ¼ cup flour
- 3 eggs
- 1 cup panko bread crumbs

- ½ cup brown sugar
- 1/3 cup red hot sauce
- ½ teaspoon garlic powder
- 3 tablespoons water

Directions:
1. Preheat the 425⁰F.
2. Cut the chicken breasts into strips.
3. Place the chicken in a Ziploc bag and add the flour. Shake to coat.
4. Place the bread crumbs in a bowl.
5. Place the egg in another bowl.
6. Dip the floured meat into the eggs then into the breadcrumbs.
7. Place the chicken on a baking sheet and spray with cooking oil on top.
8. Bake in the oven for 20 minutes.
9. Meanwhile, make the sauce by mixing the remaining Ingredients: in a saucepan.
10. Serve the chicken tenders with the meat.

Chicken Fried Rice

Servings Per Recipe: 6, POINTS:2
Cooking Time: 12 minutes

Ingredients:
- 1 teaspoon olive oil
- 4 large egg whites
- 1 onion, chopped
- 2 cloves of garlic, minced
- 12 ounces skinless chicken breasts, cut into ½" cubes
- ½ cups carrots, chopped
- ½ cup frozen green peas
- 2 cups long-grain brown rice, cooked
- 3 tablespoons soy sauce, low-sodium

Directions:
1. Coat a skillet with oil and heat over medium high flame.

2. Add the egg whites and cook until scrambled. Set aside.
3. Sauté the onions, garlic, and chicken breasts for 6 minutes until lightly brown.
4. Add the carrots and green peas. Continue cooking for another 3 minutes.
5. Stir in the rice and season with soy sauce.
6. Add the cooked egg whites and stir for 3 more minutes.

Irresistible Potato and Cheese Casserole

Ingredients:
- Salt
- Pepper
- 4 beaten eggs
- 1 can milk, evaporated
- 3 oz. bacon, chopped
- ½ c. scallion, sliced
- 3 c. potato, shredded
- ¾ c. cheddar cheese

Directions:
1. For this recipe, turn on the oven and let it heat up to 350 degrees. Take out your baking pan and coat it with some cooking spray.
2. Place the potatoes into the prepared baking pan and then top with some cheese, scallions, and bacon.
3. Now bring out a small bowl and mix together the pepper, salt, eggs, and milk inside. Pour this all on top of the potato mixture.
4. Place this meal inside the oven and let it cook for 40 minutes or until everything has time to set.
5. Take it out of the oven and give it a few minutes to cool down before slicing and enjoying.

Freestyle Soup Recipes
Chicken & Veggie Soup

(Prep Time 20 mins | Cooking Time 25 mins)

Ingredients:
- 2 tablespoons olive oil
- 1 large onion, chopped
- 2 zucchinis, chopped
- 2 large potatoes, peeled and chopped
- 4 parsnips, peeled and chopped
- 1 cup fresh peas, shelled
- 16-ounce chicken breasts
- 2 teaspoons ground cumin
- 1 tablespoon ground turmeric
- 4 cups chicken broth
- 6 cups water

Instructions:
1. In a large soup pan, heat oil over medium heat and sauté onion for about 3 minutes.
2. Stir in vegetables and cook for about 5 minutes. Stir in remaining ingredients and bring to a boil.
3. Reduce the heat to medium-low and simmer for about 10-15 minutes.
4. Remove the chicken breasts from soup and with 2 forks, shred them.
5. Return the shredded chicken into soup and simmer for about 10 minutes. Serve hot.

Servings | 10   Per portion: Calories | 211   Fat | 6.2g   Protein | 15.3g   Carbohydrates | 24g
Freestyle: 6 points

Cod & Quinoa Soup

(Prep Time 20 mins | Cooking Time 1 hour)

Ingredients:
- 2 cups onions, chopped
- 1 cup celeriac root, chopped
- 2 garlic cloves, chopped
- 2 tablespoons fresh ginger, chopped finely
- 1 cup shiitake mushrooms, sliced
- 1 cup quinoa
- 4 cups vegetable broth
- 4 cups water
- 14-ounce cod fillets
- 6 cups fresh baby spinach
- 1 cup fresh cilantro, chopped
- 1 cup unsweetened almond milk
- Salt and ground black pepper, to taste
- 2 scallions, chopped

Instructions:
1. In a large pan, add onions, celeriac root, garlic, ginger root, mushrooms, quinoa and broth and bring to a boil.
2. Reduce the heat to low and simmer, covered for about 45 minutes. Arrange the halibut fillets over soup mixture and simmer, covered for about 15 minutes.
3. Stir in remaining ingredients except scallions and simmer for about 5 minutes.
4. Serve hot with the garnishing of scallions.

Servings| 8   Per portion: Calories| 200   Fat| 3.1g   Protein| 12.9g   Carbohydrates| 31.2g

Freestyle: 5 points

Chicken & Lime Soup

(Prep Time 20 mins | Cooking Time 8 hours)

Ingredients:
- 2 cups boneless chicken, cubed
- 1 small onion, chopped
- 4 garlic cloves, minced
- 6-ounce mushrooms, chopped
- 1 medium tomato chopped
- 4 cups chicken broth
- ¼ cup fresh lime juice
- ½ teaspoon dried oregano
- ½ teaspoon ground cumin
- ½ teaspoon red chili powder
- Salt and freshly ground black pepper, to taste

Instructions:
1. In a slow cooker, add all ingredients and mix well.
2. Set the slow cooker on Low and cook, covered for about 8 hours.
3. With a slotted spoon, transfer chicken into a bowl and with 2 forks, shred it nicely.
4. Transfer the chicken into soup and stir to combine. Serve immediately.

Servings| 5   Per portion: Calories| 162 Fat| 5.5g   Protein| 21.7g Carbohydrates| 5.2g
Freestyle: 3 points

Meatballs & Kale Soup

(Prep Time 20 mins | Cooking Time 25 mins)
Ingredients:
For Meatballs:
- 1 pound lean ground turkey
- 1 garlic clove, minced
- ¼ teaspoon fresh ginger, minced
- 1 egg, beaten
- ¼ cup low-fat Parmesan cheese, grated
- Salt and ground black pepper, to taste

For Soup:
- 1 tablespoon olive oil
- 1 small onion, chopped finely
- 1 garlic clove, minced
- 1 teaspoon fresh ginger, minced
- 6 cups chicken broth
- 4 cups fresh kale, trimmed and chopped
- 2 eggs, beaten lightly
- Salt and ground black pepper, to taste

Instructions:
1. In a bowl, add all meatballs ingredients and mix until well combined. Make equal sized small balls from mixture.
2. In a large pan, heat oil over medium heat and sauté onion for about 5-6 minutes. Add garlic and ginger and sauté for about 1 minute.
3. Add broth and bring to a boil. Carefully, place the balls in pan and bring to a boil.
4. Reduce the heat to low and simmer for about 10 minutes. Stir in kale and bring the soup to a gentle simmer. Simmer for 4-5 minutes.
5. >Slowly, add beaten eggs, stirring continuously. Season with salt and black pepper and serve hot.

Servings | 6   Per portion: Calories | 246   Fat | 13.3g
Protein | 24.4g   Carbohydrates | 7.4g
Freestyle: 6 points

Beef & Veggies Soup

(Prep Time 20 mins | Cooking Time 15 mins)

Ingredients:
- 4 cups chicken broth
- 4 cups water
- 3 cups broccoli, chopped
- 8-ounce fresh mushrooms, sliced
- 2 scallions, chopped and green part reserved
- 1 (1-inch) piece fresh ginger, minced
- 5 garlic cloves, minced
- 1 pound cooked beef, sliced thinly
- ½ teaspoon red pepper flakes, crushed
- 3 tablespoons coconut aminos
- 1 lemon, sliced

Instructions:
1. In a pan, add broth and bring to a boil and cook broccoli for about 2 minutes.
2. Stir in mushroom, scallions, ginger and garlic and simmer for about 7-8 minutes.
3. Add beef, red pepper flakes and coconut aminos and stir to combine.
4. Reduce the heat to low and simmer for about 4-5 minutes.
5. Serve hot with the garnishing of reserved green part of scallion and lemon slices.

Servings | 4   Per portion: Calories | 184   Fat | 5g   Protein | 26.6g   Carbohydrates | 7g
Freestyle: 4 points

Ground Beef Soup

(Prep Time 20 mins | Cooking Time 30 mins)

Ingredients:
- 1 pound lean ground beef
- ½ pound fresh mushrooms, sliced
- 1 small onion, chopped
- 1 garlic clove, minced
- 1 teaspoon fresh ginger, minced
- 1 pound head bok choy, stalks and leaves separated and chopped
- 2 tablespoons soy sauce
- 4 cups chicken broth
- Freshly ground black pepper, to taste

Instructions:
1. Heat a large non-stick soup pan over medium-high heat and cook beef for about 5 minutes.
2. Add onion, mushrooms and garlic and cook for about 5 minutes. Add bok choy stalks and cook for about 4-5 minutes.
3. Add soy sauce and broth and bring to a boil. Reduce the heat to low and simmer, covered for about 10 minutes.
4. Stir in bok choy leaves and simmer for about 5 minutes.
5. Stir in black pepper and serve hot.

Servings | 6   Per portion: Calories | 177   Fat | 5g   Protein | 27.1g   Carbohydrates | 5.1g

Freestyle: 4 points

Meatballs & Zucchini Soup

(Prep Time 20 mins | Cooking Time 6 hours 5 mins)

Ingredients:

For Meatballs:
- 2 pounds lean ground beef
- 4 garlic cloves, minced
- ¼ cup fresh parsley, chopped
- ½ cup low-fat Parmesan cheese, grated
- 1 egg, beaten
- 1 teaspoon dried oregano
- 1 teaspoon dried rosemary
- Salt and ground black pepper, to taste
- 2 tablespoons olive oil

For Soup:
- 1 celery stalk, chopped
- 1 small onion, chopped
- 1 small carrot, peeled and chopped
- 1 large plum tomato, chopped finely
- 3 large zucchinis, spiralized with blade C
- Salt and ground black pepper, to taste
- 4 cups chicken broth
- 4 cups water

Instructions:
1. For meatballs in a large bowl, add all ingredients and mix until well combined. Make small sized balls from mixture.
2. In a large skillet, heat oil over medium-high heat and cook meatballs in batches for about 4-5 minutes or until golden brown from all sides. Remove from heat.
3. In a slow cooker, add celery, onion, carrot and tomato.
4. Place zucchini noodles over vegetables and sprinkle with salt and black pepper.
5. Pour broth over vegetables. Carefully, add meatballs in slow cooker.

6. Set the slow cooker on Low and cook, covered for about 6 hours.

Servings | 12   Per portion: Calories | 210   Fat | 10g
Protein | 24.9g   Carbohydrates | 4.9g
Freestyle: 5 points

Chicken & Zucchini Soup

(Prep Time 20 mins | Cooking Time 25 mins)
Ingredients:
- 1 tablespoon olive oil
- 1 cup carrot, peeled and chopped
- ½ cup onion, chopped
- 2 garlic cloves, minced
- 2 tablespoons fresh rosemary, chopped
- 4½ cups chicken broth
- 1¼ cups fresh spinach, torn
- 1¼ cups cooked chicken, shredded
- 1¼ cups zucchini, spiralized with Blade C
- Salt and ground black pepper, to taste
- 2 tablespoons fresh lemon juice

Instructions:
1. In a large pan, heat oil over medium heat and sauté carrots and onion for about 8-9 minutes.
2. Add garlic and rosemary and sauté for about 1 minute. Add broth and spinach and bring to a boil over high heat.
3. Reduce the heat to medium-low and simmer for about 5 minutes. Add cooked chicken and zucchini and simmer for about 5 minutes.
4. Stir in salt, black pepper and lemon juice and remove from heat. Serve hot.

Servings | 4   Per portion: Calories | 174   Fat | 6.8g
Protein | 19.5g   Carbohydrates | 8.3g
Freestyle: 4 points

Pork & Veggie Soup

(Prep Time 20 mins | Cooking Time 25 mins)

Ingredients:
- 1 tablespoon olive oil
- 1 teaspoon fresh ginger, minced
- 2 garlic cloves, minced
- ½ teaspoon dried thyme
- ½ teaspoon ground cumin
- ¼ teaspoon ground coriander
- ½ teaspoon red pepper flakes, crushed
- 1 pound lean ground pork
- Salt and ground black pepper, to taste
- 4 cups chicken broth
- 1 medium sweet potato, peeled and spiralized with Blade C
- 4 cups fresh spinach, torn
- 1 cup scallion, chopped

Instructions:
1. In a large pan, heat oil over medium heat. Add ginger, garlic, thyme and spices and sauté for about 1 minute.
2. Add pork and sprinkle with salt and black pepper and cook for about 9-10 minutes, stirring and breaking with a spoon.
3. Add broth and bring to a boil. Reduce the heat to low and simmer for about 8-10 minutes.
4. Add sweet potato and simmer for about 5 minutes. Add spinach and scallion and simmer for about 3-4 minutes.
5. Season with salt and black pepper and serve hot.

Servings | 5   Per portion: Calories | 245   Fat | 16.7g   Protein | 17.1g   Carbohydrates | 8g
Freestyle: 6 points

Salmon Soup

(Prep Time 20 mins | Cooking Time 25 mins)

Ingredients:
- 1 tablespoon olive oil
- 1 onion, chopped
- 1 garlic clove, minced
- 4 cups chicken broth
- 1 pound boneless salmon, cubed
- 1 tablespoon tamari
- 2 tablespoons fresh cilantro, chopped
- Freshly ground black pepper, to taste
- 1 tablespoon fresh lime juice

Instructions:
1. In a large soup pan, heat oil over medium heat and sauté onion for about 5 minutes.
2. Add garlic and lime leaves and sauté for about 1 minute. Add broth and bring to a boil over high heat.
3. Reduce the heat to low and simmer for about 15 minutes. Add salmon and tamari and cook for about 3-4 minutes.
4. Stir in black pepper, lime juice and cilantro and serve hot.

Servings | 5   Per portion: Calories | 209   Fat | 10.5g   Protein | 24.6g   Carbohydrates | 4.2g   Freestyle: 4 points

Veggies Soup

(Prep Time 20 mins | Cooking Time 8 hours 6 mins)

Ingredients:
- 1 tablespoon olive oil
- 1 shallot, chopped
- 2 garlic cloves, minced
- 1 medium sweet potato, peeled and chopped
- 1 zucchini, chopped
- 1 cup fresh spinach, chopped
- 1 celery stalk, chopped
- ½ cup carrot, peeled and chopped
- 2 tomatoes, chopped
- 4 cups vegetable broth
- 1 bay leaf
- ½ teaspoon dried basil
- 1 teaspoon dried oregano
- ½ teaspoon dried parsley
- Salt and ground black pepper, to taste

Instructions:
1. Set the slow cooker on high. Add oil and cook shallot and garlic for about 5-6 minutes.
2. Now, add remaining ingredients and mix well. Set the slow cooker on Low and cook, covered for about 6-8 hours.
3. Discard bay leaf and serve.

Servings | 5   Per portion: Calories | 109   Fat | 4.2g   Protein | 5.9g   Carbohydrates | 12.8g   Freestyle: 4 points

Barley & Chickpeas Soup

(Prep Time 20 mins | Cooking Time 1½ hours)

Ingredients:
- ½ cup canned chickpeas, rinsed and drained
- ½ cup dry barley
- 2 large carrots, peeled and chopped
- 1 small onion, chopped
- 1 celery stalk, chopped
- ½ (14½-ounce) can diced tomatoes with liquid
- ½ teaspoon Worcestershire sauce
- 1 teaspoon dried thyme
- 1 teaspoon curry powder
- 2 bay leaves
- Salat and ground black pepper, to taste
- 4 cups vegetable broth
- 2 tablespoons fresh parsley, chopped

Instructions:
1. In a large soup pan, add all ingredients except parsley and bring to a boil over high heat.
2. Reduce the heat to low and simmer, covered for about 1½ hours.
3. Discard bay leaf before serving. Serve hot with the garnishing of parsley.

Servings | 4   Per portion: Calories | 209   Fat | 2.3g   Protein | 8.8g   Carbohydrates | 40.5g

Freestyle: 6 points

Chicken & Greens Soup

(Prep Time 20 mins | Cooking Time 35 mins)

Ingredients:
- 1½ pound skinless, boneless chicken thighs, cut into chunks
- Salt and freshly ground black pepper, to taste
- 2 tablespoons olive oil
- 2 onions, chopped roughly
- 3 carrots, peeled and sliced
- 3 celery sticks, chopped
- 6 garlic cloves, minced
- 2 teaspoons fresh ginger, minced
- 2 teaspoons dried rosemary
- 2 teaspoons dried thyme
- 2 teaspoons ground turmeric
- 2 tablespoons apple cider vinegar
- 4 cups chicken broth
- 4½ cup water
- 6 cups green leafy vegetables (kale, Swiss chard and spinach), trimmed and chopped

Instructions:
1. Season chicken with salt and pepper evenly. In a large pan, heat oil and sear chicken for about 1-2 minutes per side. Transfer chicken into a plate.
2. In the same pan, add onion, carrots, celery, garlic and ginger and sauté for about 4-5 minutes.
3. Add herbs and spices and cook for about 2 minutes. Stir in the vinegar and scrape off the browned bits from the bottom of the pan.
4. Add the chicken broth and pieces and cook, covered for about 20 minutes. Stir in greens and cook for about 3-4 minutes.
5. Serve hot.

Servings | 8   Per portion: Calories | 180   Fat | 6.8g
Protein | 21.4g   Carbohydrates | 8.1g
Freestyle: 4 points

Rice Noodles & Veggie Soup

(Prep Time 20 mins | Cooking Time 35 mins)
Ingredients:
- 1 (3¾-ounce) package thin rice noodles
- 1 tablespoon olive oil
- 8-ounces fresh shiitake mushrooms, sliced thinly
- 2 tablespoons fresh ginger, grated
- 4 cups vegetable broth
- ¼ cup low-sodium soy sauce
- 1 teaspoon hot sauce
- 8-ounce fresh green beans, trimmed and cut into 2-inch pieces
- 2 carrots, peeled and julienned
- 2 scallions, sliced

Instructions:
1. In a large bowl, add noodles. Pour very hot water over noodles. Cover and keep aside for about 15-20 minutes or prepare according to package's directions.
2. Drain the noodles and then cut into 3-inch pieces.
3. Meanwhile in a large soup pan, heat oil over medium-high heat and cook mushrooms for about 4-5 minutes. Add ginger and sauté for about 1 minute.
4. Add broth, soy sauce and hot pepper sauce and bring to a boil. Stir in vegetables and again bring to a boil.
5. Reduce the heat to medium and simmer for about 5-7 minutes.
6. Divide noodles in serving bowls and top with hot soup. Serve immediately.

Servings| 4   Per portion: Calories| 175   Fat| 5.3g
Protein| 8.6g   Carbohydrates| 25.9g   Fat| 5.3g
Freestyle: 5 points

Snack & Appetizer Recipes

Roasted Almonds applesauce

(Prep Time 10 mins | Cooking Time 14 mins)
Ingredients:
- 2 cups whole almonds
- 3 tablespoon unsweetened applesauce
- 1 teaspoon extra-virgin olive oil
- 1 tablespoon water
- ½ teaspoon red chili powder
- ½ teaspoon ground cinnamon
- ¼ teaspoon ground cumin
- ¼ teaspoon cayenne pepper
- Salt, to taste

Instructions:
1. Preheat the oven to 350 degrees F.
2. Arrange the almonds onto a large rimmed baking sheet in a single layer. Roast for about 10 minutes.
3. Meanwhile in a microwave safe bowl, add applesauce and microwave over high for about 30 seconds. Remove from microwave and stir in oil and water. In a small bowl, mix together all spices.
4. Remove the almonds from oven. Add into the bowl of applesauce mixture and stir to combine well. Transfer the almond mixture onto baking sheet in a single layer. Sprinkle with spice mixture evenly. Roast for about 3-4 minutes.
5. Remove from oven and keep aside to cool completely before serving. You can preserve these roasted almonds in an airtight jar.

Servings | 12 Per portion: Calories | 97 Fat | 8.4g Protein | 3.4g Carbohydrates | 4g | Freestyle: 3 points

Tasty Roasted Chickpeas

(Prep Time 10 mins | Cooking Time 20 mins)
Ingredients:
- 2 cups canned chickpeas, rinsed and drained
- 1 tablespoon extra-virgin olive oil
- 1 teaspoon dried marjoram, crushed
- 1 teaspoon ground cumin
- ½ teaspoon cayenne pepper
- ¼ teaspoon ground allspice

Instructions:
1. Preheat the oven to 450 degrees F. Arrange a rack in upper third of the oven.
2. With paper towels, pat dry the chickpeas, oil, marjoram and spices and toss to coat well. Spread the chickpeas onto a rimmed baking sheet. Bake for about 25-30 minutes, stirring once in the middle way.
3. Remove from the oven and keep aide to cool on the baking sheet for about 15 minutes. You can preserve these chickpeas in an airtight jar.

Servings| 8   Per portion: Calories| 199   Fat| 4.9g
Protein|9.7g   Carbohydrates| 30.6g
Freestyle: 6 points

Hot & Spicy Popcorn

(Prep Time 15 mins | Cooking Time 5 mins)
Ingredients:
- 3 tablespoons olive oil, divided
- ½ cup popping corn
- 1 teaspoon ground turmeric
- ¼ teaspoon garlic powder
- Salt, to taste

Instructions:
1. In a pan, heat 2 tablespoons of oil over medium-high heat. Add popping corn and cover the pan tightly. Cook for about 1-2 minutes or until corn kernels start to pop, shaking the pan occasionally.

2. Remove from heat and transfer into a large heatproof bowl. Add remaining olive oil and spices and mix well. Serve immediately.

Servings | 3   Per portion: Calories | 183   Fat | 2g
Protein | 1.8g   Carbohydrates | 12.6g
Freestyle: 6 points

Salt And Pepper Spinach Chips

(Prep Time 20 mins | Cooking Time 8 mins)
Ingredients:
- 4 cups fresh spinach leaves
- 1/8 teaspoon olive oil
- ¼ teaspoon paprika
- 1/8 teaspoon ground cumin
- Salt, to taste

Instructions:
1. Preheat the oven to 325 degrees F. Line a baking sheet with a parchment paper.
2. In a large bowl, add spinach leaves and drizzle with oil. With your hands, rub the spinach leaves until all the leaves are coated with oil.
3. Sprinkle with spices and salt. Transfer the leaves onto prepared baking sheet in a single layer. Bake for about 8 minutes.
4. Serve immediately.

Servings | 2   Per portion: Calories | 18   Fat | 0.6g
Protein | 1.8g   Carbohydrates | 2.4g
Freestyle: 1 point

Bake Kale Chips

(Prep Time 20 mins | Cooking Time 15 mins)
Ingredients:
- 1 pound fresh kale leaves, stemmed and torn
- ¼ teaspoon cayenne pepper
- Salt, to taste
- 1 tablespoon olive oil

Instructions:

1. Preheat the oven to 350 degrees F. Line a large baking sheet with a parchment paper.
2. Place kale pieces into prepared baking sheet. Sprinkle the kale with salt and drizzle with oil. Bake for about 10-15 minutes.
3. Serve immediately.

Servings | 4   Per portion: Calories | 86   Fat | 3.5g
Protein | 3.4g   Carbohydrates | 11.9g
Freestyle: 2 points

Hot Pepper Apple Chips

(Prep Time 15 mins | Cooking Time 2 hours)
Ingredients:
- 2 tablespoons ground cinnamon
- 1 tablespoon ground ginger
- 1½ teaspoons ground cloves
- 1½ teaspoons ground nutmeg
- Salt and ground black pepper, to taste
- 3 Fuji apples, sliced thinly in rounds

Instructions:
1. Preheat the oven to 200 degrees F. Line a baking sheet with a parchment paper.
2. In a bowl, mix together all spices.
3. Arrange the apple slices onto prepared baking sheet in a single layer. Sprinkle the apple slices with spice mixture generously. Roast for about 1 hour.
4. Flip the side and sprinkle with spice mixture. Bake for about 1 hour.
5. Serve warm.

Servings | 6   Per portion: Calories | 71
Fat | 0.6g   Protein | 0.5g   Carbohydrates | 18.5g
Freestyle: 3 points

Ginger Parsnip Fries

(Prep Time 20 mins | Cooking Time 40 mins)
Ingredients:
- 2 tablespoons olive oil
- 1¼ pounds small parsnips, peeled and quartered
- 1½ tablespoons fresh ginger, minced
- ½ teaspoon chili powder
- Salt and freshly ground black pepper, to taste

Instructions:
1. Preheat the oven to 325 degrees F.
2. In a 13x9-inch baking dish, place the oil evenly.
3. Add remaining ingredients and toss to coat well. With a piece of foil, cover the baking dish and bake for about 40 minutes.
4. Serve immediately.

Servings | 4   Per portion: Calories | 174   Fat | 7.6g
Protein | 1.9g   Carbohydrates | 27.1g
Freestyle: 6 points

Roasted Pumpkin Seeds

(Prep Time 10 mins | Cooking Time 8 mins)
Ingredients:
- 1 cup pumpkin seeds, shelled
- 2 teaspoons unsweetened applesauce
- 1 teaspoon pumpkin pie spice
- ¼ teaspoon sea salt

Instructions:
1. Preheat the oven to 350 degrees F. Line a baking sheet with a piece of foil.
2. In a bowl, add all ingredients and toss to coat well. Spread the seeds onto prepared baking sheet in a single layer. Bake for about 8 minutes.
3. Remove from oven and keep aside to cool completely. You can store these seeds in an airtight container.

Servings | 6   Per portion: Calories | 126 Fat | 10.6g
Protein | 5.7g   Carbs | 4.5g | Freestyle: 4 points

Roasted Cashews

(Prep Time 10 mins | Cooking Time 20 mins)
Ingredients:
- 2 cups cashews
- 2 teaspoon unsweetened applesauce
- 1½ teaspoon smoked paprika
- ½ teaspoon chili flakes
- Pinch of salt
- 1 tablespoon fresh lemon juice
- 1 teaspoon olive oil

Instructions:
1. Preheat the oven to 350 degrees F. Line a baking dish with the parchment paper.
2. In a bowl, add all ingredients and toss to coat well. Transfer the cashew mixture into prepared baking dish in a single layer. Roast for about 20 minutes, flipping once in the middle way.
3. Remove from oven and keep aside to cool completely before serving. You can preserve these roasted cashews in an airtight jar.

Servings | 12   Per portion: Calories | 136   Fat | 11g
Protein | 3.6g   Carbohydrates | 7.7g
Freestyle: 5 points

Russet Potato Fries

(Prep Time 20 mins | Cooking Time 10 mins)
Ingredients:
- 1 large russet potato, peeled and cut into 1/8-inch thick sticks lengthwise
- ¼ teaspoon ground turmeric
- ¼ teaspoon red chili powder
- Salt, to taste
- 1 tablespoon olive oil

Instructions:
1. Preheat the oven to 400 degrees F. Line 2 baking sheets with parchment papers.

2. In a large bowl, add all ingredients and toss to coat well. Transfer the mixture into prepared baking sheets in a single layer. Bake for about 10 minutes.
3. Serve immediately.

Servings | 2   Per portion: Calories | 208   Fat | 7.2g
Protein | 4g   Carbohydrates | 33.7g
Freestyle: 6 points

Cauliflower Poppers

(Prep Time 20 mins | Cooking Time 30 mins)

Ingredients:
- 4 cups cauliflower florets
- 2 teaspoons olive oil
- ¼ teaspoon red chili powder
- Salt and freshly ground black pepper, to taste

Instructions:
1. Preheat the oven to 450 degrees F. Grease a roasting pan.
2. In a bowl, add all ingredients and toss to coat well. Transfer the mixture into prepared roasting pan. Roast for about 25-30 minutes.
3. Serve warm.

Servings | 4   Per portion: Calories | 46   Fat | 2.5g
Protein | 2g   Carbohydrates | 5.4g
Freestyle: 2 points

Quinoa Croquettes

(Prep Time 20 mins | Cooking Time 16 mins)

Ingredients:
- ¼ cup plus 1 tablespoon olive oil, divided
- ½ cup frozen peas, thawed
- 2 garlic cloves, minced
- 1 cup cooked quinoa
- 2 large boiled potatoes, peeled and mashed
- ¼ cup fresh cilantro, chopped
- 2 teaspoons ground cumin
- ½ teaspoon paprika
- ¼ teaspoon ground turmeric

- Salt and freshly ground black pepper, to taste

Instructions:
1. In a frying pan, heat 1 tablespoon of oil over medium heat and sauté peas and garlic for about 1 minute.
2. Transfer the peas mixture into a large bowl. Add remaining ingredients and mix until well combined. Make equal sized oblong shaped patties from the mixture.
3. In a large skillet, heat remaining oil over medium-high heat. Add croquettes in batches and fry for about 4 minutes per side.
4. Serve warm.

Servings | 12   Per portion: Calories | 120   Fat | 5.2g
Protein | 3.1g   Carbohydrates | 16g
Freestyle: 4 points

Coconut Chicken Popcorn

(Prep Time 20 mins | Cooking Time 25 mins)

Ingredients:
- ½ pound boneless chicken thigh, cut into bite-sized pieces
- 7-ounce unsweetened almond milk
- 1 teaspoons ground turmeric
- Salt and freshly ground black pepper, to taste
- 2 tablespoons coconut flour
- 3 tablespoons desiccated coconut
- 1 tablespoon olive oil

Instructions:
1. In a large bowl, mix together chicken, coconut milk, turmeric, salt and black pepper. Refrigerate, covered overnight.
2. Preheat the oven to 390 degrees F.
3. In a shallow dish, mix together coconut flour and desiccated coconut. Coat the chicken pieces with coconut mixture evenly.

4. Arrange chicken piece onto a baking sheet and drizzle with oil evenly. Bake for about 20-25 minutes.
   5. Serve warm.

Servings | 4   Per portion: Calories | 169   Protein | 17.1g   Carbohydrates | 3.5g   Fat | 9.4g
Freestyle: 4 points

Butter Currant Biscuits

(Prep Time 20 mins | Cooking Time 15 mins)

Ingredients:
- 2 cups flour
- 1 teaspoon baking powder
- ¼ teaspoon salt
- 4 tablespoons butter
- 5 tablespoons milk
- ½ cup currants

Instructions:
1. Preheat the oven to 400 degrees F. Grease a baking sheet.
2. In a bowl, sift together flour, baking powder and salt. Add in butter and mix until a coarse cornmeal like mixture is formed. Add milk and currants and mix until a soft dough is formed.
3. Place the dough onto a lightly floured surface and roll into ½-inch thickness. With a biscuit cutter, cut ½-inch of circles.
4. Arrange circles onto prepared baking sheet in a single layer. Bake for about 15 minutes.

Servings | 10   Per portion: Calories | 138   Fat | 4.9g   Protein | 3g   Carbohydrates | 20.5g
Freestyle: 5 points

Green Deviled Eggs

(Prep Time 15 mins | Cooking Time 20 mins)
Ingredients:
- 6 large eggs
- 1 medium avocado, peeled, pitted and chopped
- 2 teaspoons fresh lime juice
- Pinch of salt
- 1/8 teaspoon cayenne pepper

Instructions:
1. In a pan of water, add eggs and cook for about 15-20 minutes. Drain the water and let the eggs cool completely. Peel the eggs and with a sharp knife, slice them in half vertically. Scoop out the yolks and transfer half of them into a bowl.
2. In the bowl of yolks, add avocado, lime juice and salt and with a fork, mash until well combined. Fill the egg halves with avocado mixture. Sprinkle with cayenne pepper and serve.

Servings | 6   Per portion: Calories | 140   Fat | 11.5g   Protein | 6.9g   Carbohydrates | 3.3g
Freestyle: 4 points

Tomato Bruschetta

(Prep Time 20 mins | Cooking Time 4 mins)
Ingredients:
- ½ of whole-grain baguette, cut into 6 (½-inch-thick) slices diagonally
- 3 tomatoes, chopped
- ½ cup fennel, chopped
- 2 garlic cloves, minced
- 1 tablespoon fresh parsley, chopped
- 1 tablespoon fresh basil, chopped
- 2 teaspoons balsamic vinegar
- 1 teaspoon olive oil
- Salt and ground black pepper, to taste

Instructions:

1. Preheat the oven to broiler. Arrange a rack in the top portion of the oven.
2. Arrange the bread slices onto a baking sheet in a single layer. Broil for about 2 minutes per side.
3. Meanwhile in a bowl, add remaining ingredients and toss to coat. Place the tomato mixture on each toasted bread slice evenly and serve immediately.

Servings | 6   Per portion: Calories | 24 Fat | 0.9g
Protein | 0.8g   Carbohydrates | 3.7g
Freestyle: 1 points

Vanilla Almond Scones

(Prep Time 20 mins | Cooking Time 20 mins)
Ingredients:
- 1 cup almonds
- 1 1/3 cups almond flour
- ¼ cup arrowroot flour
- 1 tablespoon coconut flour
- 1 teaspoon ground turmeric
- Salt and ground black pepper, to taste
- 1 egg
- ¼ cup olive oil
- 3 tablespoons unsweetened applesauce
- 1 teaspoon vanilla extract

Instructions:
1. Preheat the oven to 350 degrees F.
2. In a food processor, add almonds and pulse until chopped roughly. Transfer the chopped almonds in a large bowl.
3. Add flours and spices and mix well. In another bowl, add remaining ingredients and beat until well combined.
4. Add flour mixture into egg mixture and mix until well combined.
5. Arrange a plastic wrap over cutting board. Place the dough over cutting board. With your hands, pat into about 1-inch thick circle.

6. Carefully, cut the circle in 7 wedges. Arrange the scones onto a cookie sheet in a single layer.
7. Bake for about 15-20 minutes.

Servings | 7   Per portion: Calories | 192   Fat | 17.4g
Protein | 5.2g   Carbohydrates | 6.4g
Freestyle: 6 points

Blueberry Balls Cookie

(Prep Time 20 mins)

Ingredients:
- 1 scoop unsweetened protein powder
- ½ cup coconut flour, sifted
- 1-2 tablespoons Swerve
- ¼ teaspoon ground cinnamon
- Pinch of salt
- ¼ cup dried blueberries
- ½-1 cup unsweetened almond milk

Instructions:
1. Line a large cookie sheet with parchment paper. Keep aside.
2. In a large bowl, mix together all ingredients except almond milk.
3. Slowly, add desired amount of almond milk and mix until a dough is formed. Immediately, make desired sized balls from mixture.
4. Arrange the balls onto prepared baking sheet in a single layer. Refrigerate to set for about 30 minutes before serving.

Servings | 8   Per portion: Calories | 56   Fat | 1.3g
Protein | 4.2g   Carbohydrates | 7.1g
Freestyle: 2 points

In the next section, I've included my favorite recipes that I could recommend, Although, points is of the old smart points system but never the less still usable and as tasty as always, so let enjoy!

Bonus The Best Smart Points Main course Recipes

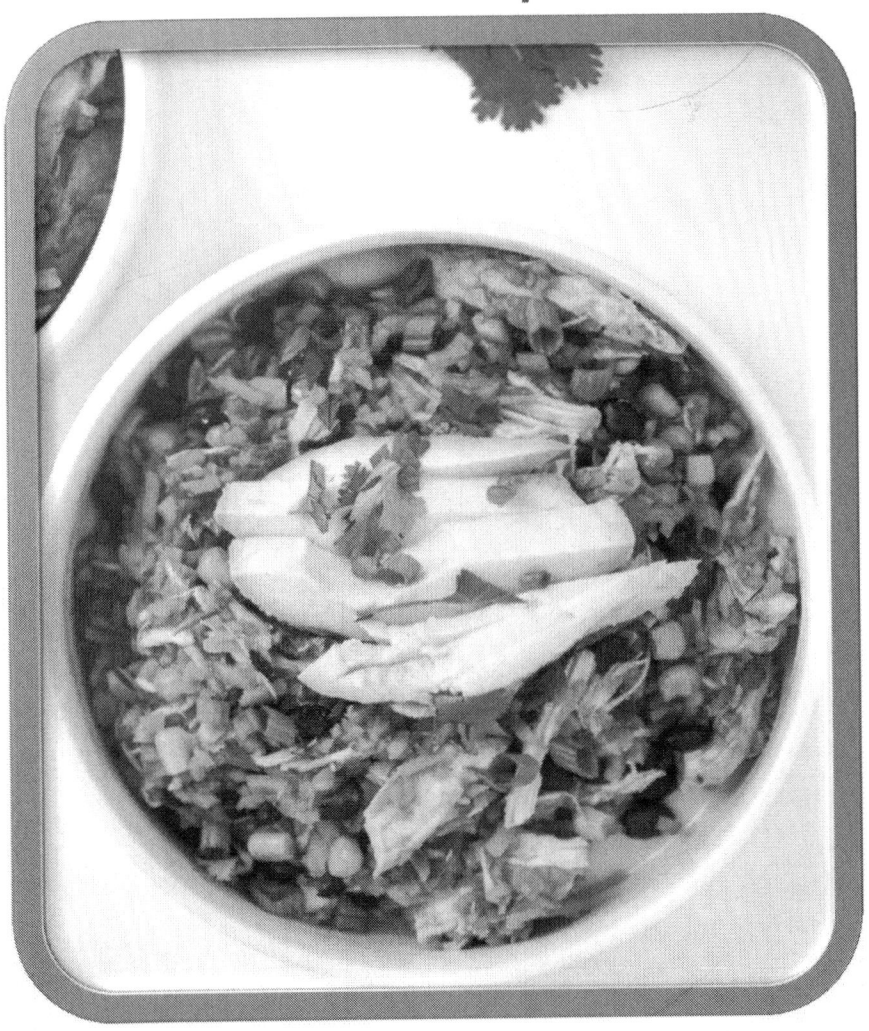

Honey Sesame Chicken

Serves: 4
6 SmartPoints™

Ingredients:

1 pound boneless, skinless chicken breast
2 teaspoons coconut oil
½ teaspoon salt
1 teaspoon coarse ground black pepper
½ teaspoon cayenne powder
1 tablespoon freshly grated ginger
2 tablespoons honey
¼ cup soy sauce
2 teaspoons sesame oil
1 tablespoon sesame seeds, toasted (optional)
Fresh lemongrass for garnish, optional
Cooked rice for serving (optional)

Directions:

1. Using a meat mallet, flatten the chicken until it is approximately ¼ inch thick.
2. Melt the coconut oil in a skillet over medium heat.
3. Season the chicken with salt, black pepper, and cayenne powder. Cook the chicken in the skillet for 4-5 minutes per side, or until it is no longer pink in the center.
4. In a small bowl, combine the fresh ginger, honey, soy sauce, and sesame oil. Mix well and pour the sauce over the chicken.

Chicken Fried Rice

Serves: 4
4 SmartPoints™

Ingredients:
4 large egg whites
12 ounces boneless, skinless chicken breast, cut in ½-inch pieces
½ cup carrot, diced
½ cup scallion (green and white parts), chopped
2 garlic cloves, minced
½ cup frozen green peas, thawed
2 cups cooked brown rice, hot
3 tablespoons soy sauce (low-sodium)

Directions:
1. Coat a large, nonstick skillet with cooking spray, and set it over medium-high heat.
2. Add the egg whites and stir frequently as you cook, until they are scrambled, about 3-5 minutes. Place the eggs on a plate and set them aside.
3. Remove the pan from the heat and coat it again with cooking spray and place it over medium-high heat.
4. Add the chicken and carrots and sauté for about 5 minutes or until the chicken is golden brown. Check that the chicken is cooked through before adding the other ingredients.
5. When the chicken is ready, add the chopped scallions, minced garlic, peas, cooked brown rice, the egg whites, and soy sauce. Stir until the ingredients have combined well and continue cooking until all the ingredients are well heated.
6. Serve and enjoy.

Nutritional Information:
Calories 178, Total Fat 2.0 g, Saturated Fat 0.8 g, Total Carbohydrate 21.0 g, Dietary Fiber 38.0 g, Sugars 2.0 g, Protein 18.0 g

Tasty Orange Chicken

Serves: 4
3 SmartPoints™

Ingredients:
2 teaspoons olive oil or cooking spray
¾ cup sweet yellow onion, sliced
1 cup red bell pepper, sliced
1 pound boneless, skinless chicken breast, cubed
½ teaspoon salt
1 teaspoon coarse ground black pepper
1 teaspoon garlic powder
¼ cup low sugar orange marmalade
2 tablespoons soy sauce
Cooked rice for serving (optional)

Directions:
1. Heat the olive oil or cooking spray in a skillet over medium heat.
2. Place the onion and red bell pepper in the skillet and cook for 3-5 minutes, or until the vegetables are just starting to become tender. Remove from the skillet and set aside.
3. Season the chicken with the salt, black pepper and garlic powder. Add the chicken to the skillet and cook, stirring occasionally, for 5-7 minutes.
4. While the chicken is cooking, combine the marmalade and soy sauce. Mix well and then add to the chicken. Toss to coat.
5. Add the vegetables back into the skillet and continue to cook for an additional 5-7 minutes, or until the chicken is cooked through.
6. Remove from the heat and serve warm with cooked rice, if desired.

Nutritional Information:
Calories 173, Total Fat 3.1 g, Saturated Fat 0.8 g, Total Carbohydrate 8.4 g, Dietary Fiber 0.9 g, Sugars 4.6 g, Protein 26.4 g

Cajun Chicken and Sweet Potato Hash

Serves: 4
5 SmartPoints™

Ingredients:
2 teaspoons olive oil or cooking spray
4 cups sweet potatoes, peeled and shredded
1 cup sweet yellow onion, diced
1 cup red bell pepper, diced
1 teaspoon salt
1 teaspoon black pepper
1 teaspoon Cajun seasoning mix
2 cups boneless skinless chicken breast, cooked and shredded
2 cups tomatoes, chopped
Fresh scallions, sliced for garnish (optional)

Directions:
1. Heat the olive oil or cooking spray in a large skillet over medium-high heat.
2. In a bowl, combine the sweet potatoes, onion, and red bell pepper. Toss to mix.
3. Add the vegetable mixture to the skillet and cook for 5-7 minutes, stirring frequently.
4. Season the vegetables with salt, black pepper and Cajun seasoning. Using a spatula, press the vegetables firmly into the bottom of the pan. Reduce the heat to medium and let them cook, without disturbing them, for 5-7 minutes, or until a crust begins to form on the bottom of the vegetables.

Spiced Pork with Apples

Serves: 6
5 SmartPoints™

Ingredients:
2 (14 ounce) pork tenderloins
Olive oil cooking spray
2 teaspoon 5-spice powder, divided
2 apples, cored and sliced
1 red onion, sliced

Directions:
1. Preheat the oven to 450°F. Remove any excess fat from the pork.
2. Line the baking pan with foil. Spray the foil lightly with olive oil cooking spray. Sprinkle 1 teaspoon 5-spice powder on the pork tenderloins and then place them on the baking pan. Roast the pork for about 20 to 30 minutes, or until it is ready.
3. Meanwhile, spray a non-stick pan with cooking spray and sauté the sliced onion until tender. Add 1 teaspoon 5-spice powder and mix well. Add the apple slices and sauté again until the mixture becomes soft and the onions are cooked. Cut the pork tenderloins into ½-inch slices and top them with the apple and onion mixture. Serve.

Nutritional Information:
Calories 253, Total Fat 9.3 g, Saturated Fat 3.2 g, Total Carbohydrate 9.2 g, Dietary Fiber 1.7 g, Sugars 4.1 g, Protein 31.9 g

Pork Chops with Salsa

Serves: 4
4 SmartPoints™

Ingredients:
4 ounces boneless pork loin chops (lean), trimmed
Cooking spray
⅓ Cup salsa
2 tablespoons lime juice, freshly squeezed
¼ cup fresh cilantro or parsley, chopped

Directions:
1. Place the chops on a flat surface and press each one of them with the palm of your hand to flatten them slightly.
2. Coat a large, nonstick skillet with cooking spray. Place it over high heat until the oil becomes hot. Add the chops to the skillet and cook each side for 1 minute, or until they are colored medium-brown. Reduce the heat to medium-low.
3. Mix the salsa and the fresh lime juice together and pour the mixture over the chops. Simmer, uncovered for about 8 minutes or until the chops are cooked through.
4. Garnish the chops with chopped cilantro or parsley (if desired). Serve.

Nutritional Information:
Calories 184, Total Fat 8.0 g, Saturated Fat 12.0 g, Total Carbohydrate 2.0 g, Sugars 0.6 g, Protein 25.0 g

Italian Steak Rolls

Serves: 4
5 SmartPoints™

Ingredients:
1 pound flank steak, thinly sliced in sheets
¼ cup low fat Italian salad dressing
1 cup red bell pepper, sliced
½ pound asparagus spears, trimmed
1 cup onion, sliced
Cooking spray
1 teaspoon salt
1 teaspoon black pepper
Kitchen twine

Directions:
1. Place the steaks in a bowl and cover them with the Italian salad dressing. Toss to coat. Set aside for 15 minutes.
2. Preheat the oven to 350°F and line a baking sheet with aluminum foil.
3. Remove the meat from the marinade and lay the slices out on a flat surface. Season with salt and black pepper as desired.
4. Place the red bell pepper, asparagus and onion pieces on the center of each piece of meat in equal amounts.
5. Roll up each piece of meat around the vegetables and secure with kitchen twine.
6. Heat the cooking spray in a skillet over medium high.
7. Add the steak rolls to the skillet and sear on all sides.
7. Transfer the steak rolls to the baking sheet. Place it in the oven and bake for 15-20 minutes, or until the meat is cooked through and the vegetables are crisp tender.
8. Remove from the oven and let rest 5 minutes before serving.

Beef Soba Bowls

Serves: 4
8 SmartPoints™

Ingredients:
1 pound flank or skirt steak, thinly sliced
Cooking spray
1 teaspoon salt
1 teaspoon black pepper
1 teaspoon ground ginger
4 cups fresh snow peas, washed and trimmed
¼ cup soy sauce
1 cup beef stock
½ pound soba noodles, cooked
Fresh cilantro for garnish (optional)
Lime wedges for garnish (optional)

Directions:
1. Spray a large skillet with vegetable oil and heat over medium.
2. Add the steak slices and season with salt, black pepper, and ground ginger. Cook, stirring occasionally, for 5-7 minutes, or until the meat has reached the desired doneness.
3. Remove the steak from the pan and keep it warm.
4. Add the snow peas to the pan and sauté for 2-3 minutes.
5. Combine the beef stock and soy sauce and add them to the skillet. Cook for 2-3 minutes, or until the liquid comes to a low boil.
6. Add the cooked soba noodles and toss. Cook an additional 1-2 minutes, or until warmed through.
7. Transfer the noodles, broth, and snow peas to a serving bowl and top with slices of steak.
8. Garnish with fresh cilantro and lime wedges before serving, if desired.

Baked Artichoke Chicken

Serves: 4
3 SmartPoints™

Ingredients:
1 pound chicken breast tenders
Cooking spray
1 teaspoon salt
1 teaspoon coarse ground black pepper
1 cup jarred artichoke hearts
1 cup heirloom tomatoes, chopped
3 cloves garlic, crushed and minced
½ cup fresh basil, torn
1 tablespoon olive oil

Directions:
1. Preheat the oven to 375°F and spray an 8x8 or larger baking dish.
2. Place the chicken tenders in an even layer in the baking dish and season with the salt and coarse ground black pepper.
3. Combine the artichoke hearts, tomatoes, garlic, and basil in a bowl. Drizzle in the olive oil and toss to mix.
4. Spread the artichoke mixture over the chicken.
5. Place in the oven and bake for 25-30 minutes, or until the chicken is cooked through.
6. Remove from the oven and let rest at least 5 minutes before serving.

Nutritional Information: *Calories 185, Total Fat 3.2 g, Saturated Fat 0.8 g, Total Carbohydrate 8.9 g, Dietary Fiber 2.0 g, Sugars 1.5 g, Protein 28.4 g*

Slow Cooker Spiced Pulled Pork

Serves 6
5 SmartPoints™

Ingredients

<u>Rub</u>
1 tablespoon paprika
1-3 teaspoons ancho chili powder according to taste
1 teaspoon salt
1 teaspoon ground cumin
1 teaspoon dry oregano
½ teaspoon black pepper
¼ teaspoon cinnamon
¼ teaspoon dry coriander

<u>Other ingredients</u>
2 pounds pork tenderloin, trimmed
1 onion, diced
4 garlic cloves, minced
1 cup low fat beef broth
1 tablespoon apple cider vinegar

Directions

1. Mix together all the rub ingredients in a small bowl.
2. Rub the spice mix all over the pork
3. Place the garlic, onion, beef broth and apple cider vinegar in the slow cooker. Stir a few times to mix well.
4. Add the pork.
5. Set on LOW and cook for 4-6 hours until the pork is cooked through and shred easily with a fork.

Nutritional Information:
Calories 190, Total Fat 4.3 g, Saturated Fat 1.2 g, Total Carbohydrate 5.4 g, Dietary Fiber 1.1 g, Sugars 0.9 g, Protein 32.8 g

Curried Pork Chops

Serves: 4
9 SmartPoints™

Ingredients:
1 pound boneless pork chops, approximately ¼ inch thick
Cooking spray
1 teaspoon salt
1 teaspoon black pepper
2 ½ cups carrots, sliced
1 cup unsweetened coconut milk
1 ½ tablespoon curry powder
1 teaspoon lime zest
Cooked rice for serving, optional

Directions:
1. Preheat the oven to 450°F and spray an 8x8 or larger baking dish with cooking spray.
2. Season the pork with salt and black pepper.
3. Place the pork and the sliced carrots in the baking dish, spreading them out into as even a layer as possible.
4. In a bowl, combine the coconut milk, curry powder, and lime zest. Mix well and pour over the pork.
5. Place the baking dish in the oven and bake for 25-30 minutes, or until the pork is cooked through and the carrots are tender.
6. Remove from the oven and let it rest for several minutes before serving.
7. Serve with cooked rice, if desired.

Nutritional Information:
Calories 367, Total Fat 20.1 g, Saturated Fat 7.5 g, Total Carbohydrate 9.9 g, Dietary Fiber 2.2 g, Sugars 3.4 g, Protein 34.9 g

Spicy Pineapple Pork

Serves: 4
8 SmartPoints™

Ingredients:
1 pound cooked pork, shredded
1 tablespoon vegetable oil or cooking spray
3 cups broccoli florets
1 teaspoon salt
1 teaspoon black pepper
2 cups medium heat tomato salsa, fresh or jarred
2 cups fresh pineapple chunks
¼ cup fresh orange juice (or other citrus juice of choice)
Fresh cilantro for serving (optional)
Cooked rice for serving (optional)

Directions:
1. Heat the vegetable oil or cooking spray in a large skillet over medium heat.
2. Add the broccoli and sauté for 5-7 minutes, or until crisp tender.
3. Add the shredded pork to the skillet and season with salt and black pepper.
4. Next, add the salsa, pineapple chunks, and orange juice. Mix well.
5. Increase the heat to medium high until the liquid comes to a low boil.
6. Reduce the heat to low, cover, and simmer for 5-7 minutes, or until heated through.
7. Remove from the heat and serve with cooked rice and cilantro, if desired.

Nutritional Information:
Calories 328, Total Fat 10.3 g, Saturated Fat 2.5 g, Total Carbohydrate 22.7 g, Dietary Fiber 5.0 g, Sugars 9.4 g, Protein 37.4 g

Breaded Veal Cutlets

Serves 4
6 SmartPoints™

Ingredients

1 pound veal cutlets, trimmed
Cooking spray
1/2 cup dry whole-wheat breadcrumbs
1/2 teaspoon paprika
1/2 teaspoon onion powder
1/2 teaspoon salt and black pepper
4 teaspoons canola oil
1 large egg white
4 teaspoons cornstarch

Directions

1. Pound the veal cutlet if needed, so they are ½ inch thick.
2. Preheat oven to 400°F. And line a rimmed baking sheet with parchment paper. Spray lightly with cooking spray.
3. Mix breadcrumbs, and spices in a shallow bowl. Add the oil and mix well.
4. Sprinkle cornstarch over the veal cutlets to evenly coat both sides.
5. Beat the egg white until it becomes frothy. Place in a shallow dish.
6. Add the veal cutlets to the egg white. Massage to coat. Add the cutlets one by one to the breadcrumbs and spices mixt. Try to coat as evenly as possible.
7. Arrange the veal cutlets on the baking sheet. Bake in the preheated oven for 15to 18 minutes, until golden and cooked through.

Nutritional Information:

Calories 219, Total Fat 7 g, Saturated Fat 2.7 g, Total Carbohydrate 11.2 g, Dietary Fiber 1.1 g, Sugars 1.7 g, Protein 24.8 g

Cheesy Fajita Casserole

Serves: 4
5 SmartPoints™

Ingredients:
½ teaspoon salt
1 teaspoon coarse ground black pepper
1 teaspoon cumin
½ teaspoon cayenne powder
½ teaspoon smoked paprika
Cooking spray
1 pound chicken breast tenders
2 cups yellow and green bell peppers, sliced
1 cup red onion, sliced
1 cup stewed tomatoes, chopped, juice included
¾ cup queso fresco cheese, crumbled
Fresh cilantro for garnish (optional)

Directions:
1. Combine the salt, black pepper, cumin, cayenne powder and smoked paprika. Set aside.
2. Preheat the oven to 375°F and spray an 8x8 or larger baking dish with cooking spray.
3. Arrange the chicken tenders in an even layer in the baking dish and season liberally with at least half of the seasoning mixture.
4. Place the bell peppers and onions over the chicken, followed by the stewed tomatoes.
5. Add any remaining seasoning mixture to the top of the peppers and onions.
6. Sprinkle the queso fresco cheese over the top and place the pan in the oven.
7. Bake uncovered for 25-30 minutes, or until the chicken is cooked through.
8. Remove from the oven and let sit for 5 minutes.
9. Serve warm, garnished with fresh cilantro, if desired.

Creamy Dijon Chicken

Serves: 4
3 SmartPoints™

Ingredients:
1 pound boneless, skinless chicken breasts
1 tablespoon olive oil or cooking spray
1 teaspoon salt
1 teaspoon white pepper
1 teaspoon fresh thyme
¼ cup Dijon mustard
½ cup low fat milk
2 cloves garlic, crushed and minced
4 cups fresh spinach, torn

Directions:
1. Heat the olive oil in a skillet over medium heat.
2. Using a meat mallet, pound the chicken until it reaches a thickness of approximately ¼ inch.
3. Season the chicken with salt, white pepper and fresh thyme. Add the chicken to the skillet and cook for 3-4 minutes per side.
4. Combine the Dijon mustard, milk, and garlic.
5. Add the Dijon mixture to the skillet and cook for 1-2 minutes.
6. Add the spinach and cook an additional 4-5 minutes, turning the chicken occasionally, until the chicken is cooked through and the spinach is wilted.
7. Remove from heat and serve warm with favorite accompaniment.

Nutritional Information:
Calories 170, Total Fat 3.2 g, Saturated Fat 0.8 g, Total Carbohydrate 2.6 g, Dietary Fiber 0.7 g, Sugars 1.7 g, Protein 27.6 g

Grilled Chicken Salad

Serves: 4
6 SmartPoints™

Ingredients:

¼ cup mayonnaise (low-fat)
1 teaspoon curry powder
2 teaspoons water
4 ounces or 1 cup rotisserie chicken, preferably lemon herb flavor, chopped
¾ cup apple, chopped
⅓ Cup celery, diced
3 tablespoons raisins
⅛ Teaspoon salt

Directions:

1. In a medium-sized bowl, combine the mayonnaise, curry powder, and water. Stir with a whisk until well blended.
2. Add the chopped chicken, celery, raisins, chopped apple, and salt. Stir the ingredients so they get combined well. Cover the salad and chill in the fridge. Serve in a lettuce wrap, with bread, or on its own.

Nutritional Information:

Calories 222, Total Fat 5.4 g, Saturated Fat 2.1 g, Total Carbohydrate 26.9 g, Dietary Fiber 2.5 g, Sugars 8.1 g, Protein 23.0 g

Delicious Chicken Salad

Serves: 4
4 SmartPoints™

Ingredients:
2 ½ cups chicken, cooked and chopped
3 stalks celery, chopped
1 cup apple, chopped
¼ cup cranberries, dried
½ cup plain Greek yogurt (nonfat)
2 tablespoons Hellman's mayonnaise, light
2 teaspoons lemon juice
Salt and pepper to taste

<u>Optional:</u>
2 tablespoons fresh parsley, chopped

Directions:
1. In a large bowl, mix the chicken, celery, apple, and dried cranberries. Stir the ingredients and combine them well.
2. In a small bowl, mix the yogurt, mayonnaise, and lemon juice. Add the mixture to the chicken mixture and mix well. Stir in the chopped parsley, if using. Add salt and pepper to taste.
3. Serve on whole grain crackers, rice, pita bread, or make a wrap.

Nutritional Information:
Calories 220 Total Fat 5.0 g, Saturated Fat 1.1 g, Total Carbohydrate 13.0 g, Dietary Fiber 2.0 g, Sugars 7.1 g, Protein 28.0 g

Raspberry Balsamic Chicken

Serves: 3
5 SmartPoints™

Ingredients:
3 pieces boneless skinless chicken breast
¼ cup all-purpose flour
Cooking spray
⅔ Cup chicken broth (low fat)
½ cup raspberry preserve (low sugar)
1 ½ teaspoons cornstarch
1 ½ tablespoons balsamic vinegar
Salt and black pepper to taste

Directions:
1. Cut the boneless and skinless chicken breast into bite-sized pieces. (You may also pound them into thin cutlets to cook through easily.) Season the chicken with salt and black pepper to taste. Dredge the chicken pieces in the flour, and shake off any excess.
2. Heat a non-stick skillet over medium heat and coat it with spray. Cook the chicken for about 15 minutes, turning halfway through so both sides can cook well. Remove the cooked chicken from the skillet.
3. Mix the chicken broth, raspberry preserves, and cornstarch in the skillet over medium heat. Stir in the balsamic vinegar. Add chicken back to the pan. Cook for about 10 minutes, turning halfway through.

Nutritional Information:
Calories 229, Total Fat 4. 6 g, Saturated Fat 0.8 g, Total Carbohydrate 21.8 g, Dietary Fiber 0.7 g, Sugars 15.0 g, Protein 24.5 g

Thank for making it through to the end of *this book*. Let's hope it was informative and able to provide you with all of the tools you need to achieve your weight loss goals. The next step is to get to the kitchen for preparing the delicious meals. Good Luck